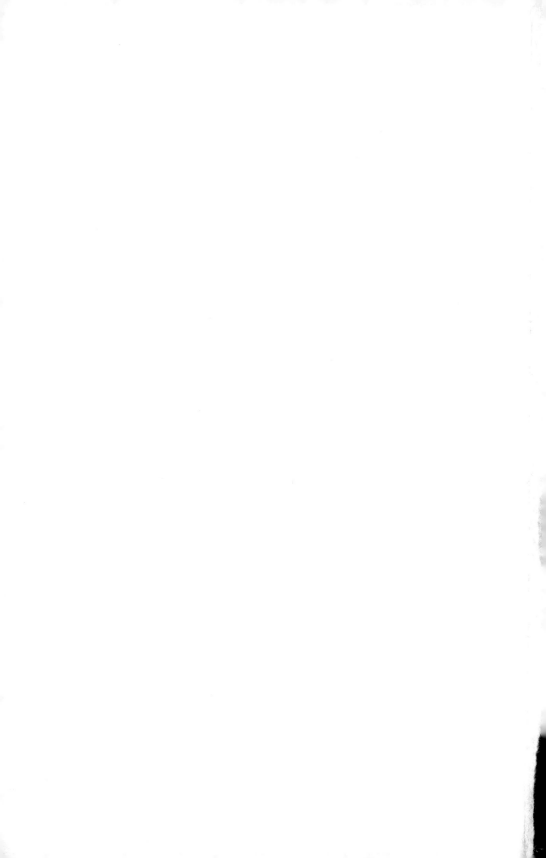

Prostate Cancer: A Multidisciplinary Guide

Prostate Cancer: A Multidisciplinary Guide

Edited by

Philip W. Kantoff, M.D.
Medical Oncology
Director, Genitourinary Oncology,
Dana-Farber Cancer Institute
Harvard Medical School
Boston, Massachusetts

Kenneth I. Wishnow, M.D.
Urology
New England Deaconess Hospital,
Harvard Medical School
Boston, Massachusetts

Kevin R. Loughlin, M.D.
Urology
Brigham and Women's Hospital
Harvard Medical School
Boston, Massachusetts

b

Blackwell
Science

Blackwell Science

Editorial offices:

350 Main Street, Malden, Massachusetts 02148, USA

Osney Mead, Oxford OX2 0El, England

25 John Street, London WC1N 2BL, England

23 Ainslie Place, Edinburgh EH3 6AJ, Scotland

54 University Street, Carlton, Victoria 3053, Australia

Other Editorial Offices:

Arnette Blackwell SA, 224, Boulevard Saint Germain, 75007 Paris, France

Blackwell Wissenschafts-Verlag GmbH Kurfürstendamm 57, 10707 Berlin, Germany Zehetnergasse 6, A-1140 Vienna, Austria

Distributors:

USA

Blackwell Science, Inc.
Commerce Place
350 Main Street
Malden, Massachusetts 02148
(Telephone orders: 800-215-1000 or 617-388-8250; Fax orders: 617-388-8270)

Canada

Copp Clark Professional
200 Adelaide Street, West, 3rd Floor
Toronto, Ontario M5H 1W7
(Telephone orders: 416-597-1616
1-800-815-9417
fax: 416-597-1617

Australia

Blackwell Science Pty., Ltd.
54 University Street
Carlton, Victoria 3053
(Telephone orders: 03-9347-0300; fax orders 03-9349 3016)

Outside North America and Australia

Blackwell Science, Ltd.
c/o Marston Book Services, Ltd.
P.O. Box 269
Abingdon
Oxon OX14 4YN
England
(Telephone orders: 44-01235-465500;
fax orders 44-01235-465555)

Acquisitions: Christopher Davis
Production: Ellen Samia
Manufacturing: Lisa Flanagan
Typeset by Best-Set Typesetter Ltd.
Printed and bound by Bookcrafters
© 1997 by Blackwell Science, Inc.
Printed in the United States of America
97 98 99 00 5 4 3 2 1

Library of Congress Cataloging-in-Publication Data
Prostate cancer: a multidisciplinary guide/[edited by] Philip W. Kantoff, Kenneth I. Wishow, Kevin R. Loughlin.
   p. cm.
Includes bibliographical references and index.
ISBN 0-86542-456-X
1. Prostate—Cancer. I. Kantoff, Philip. II. Wishow, Kenneth I. III. Loughlin, Kevin R.
   [DNLM: 1. Prostatic Neoplasms—therapy. 2. Prostatic Neoplasms—diagnosis. 3. Prostatic Neoplasms—prevention & control. WJ 752 P96542 1996]
RC280.P7P7428   1996
616.99'463—dc21
DNLM/DC
for Library of Congress   96-39071
                                   CIP

Contents

▼   ▼   ▼   ▼   ▼   ▼   ▼   ▼

Contributors

▼　▼　▼　▼　▼　▼　▼　▼

Clair J. Beard, M.D.
Instructor,
Harvard Medical School;
Attending Physician,
Joint Center for Radiation Therapy,
Boston, Massachusetts

Glenn J. Bubley, M.D.
Associate Professor of Medicine,
Harvard Medical School,
Beth Israel Hospital,
Boston, Massachusetts

Paul A. Church, M.D.
Clinical Instructor of Surgery (Urology),
Harvard Medical School;
Staff Urologist,
New England Deaconess Hospital,
Boston, Massachusetts

Steven K. Clinton, M.D., Ph.D.
Instructor in Medicine,
Harvard Medical School;
Clinical Associate,
Dana-Farber Cancer Institute,
Boston, Massachusetts

C. Norman Coleman, M.D.
Professor of Harvard Medical School;
Chairman,
Joint Center for Radiation Therapy,
Boston, Massachusetts

Christopher L. Corless, M.D., Ph.D.
Assistant Professor of Pathology,
Oregon Health Sciences University,
Staff Pathologist,
Department of Veterans Affairs Medical Center,
Portland, Oregon

Anthony V. D'Amico, M.D., Ph.D.
Assistant Professor of Radiation Oncology,
Harvard Medical School;
Attending Radiation Oncologist,
Joint Center for Radiation Therapy,
Boston, Massachusetts

William DeWolf, M.D.
Associate Professor of Urology,
Harvard Medical School;
Urologist-in-Chief,
Beth Israel Hospital,
Boston, Massachusetts

Robert C. Eyre, M.D.
Harvard Medical School;
Division Chief, Urological Surgery,
New England Deaconess Hospital,
Boston, Massachusetts

Marc B. Garnick, M.D.
Associate Professor of Medicine,
Harvard Medical School;
Attending Physician,

Beth Israel Hospital,
Boston, Massachusetts

Philip W. Kantoff, M.D.
Medical Oncology,
Director, Genitourinary Oncology,
Dana-Farber Cancer Institute,
Harvard Medical School,
Boston, Massachusetts

Irving D. Kaplan, M.D.
Assistant Professor of Radiation Oncology,
Harvard Medical School; Attending Radiation Oncologist,
Joint Center for Radiation Therapy,
Boston, Massachusetts

Donald S. Kaufman, M.D.
Associate Clinical Professor of Medicine,
Harvard Medical School;
Physician, Medical Service,
Massachusetts General Hospital,
Boston, Massachusetts

Kerry Killbridge, M.D.
Instructor in Medicine,
Harvard Medical School;
Associate Physician,
Brigham and Women's Hospital;
Active Physician,
Dana-Farber Cancer Institute,
Boston, Massachusetts

Kevin R. Loughlin, M.D.
Urology,
Brigham and Women's Hospital,
Harvard Medical School,
Boston, Massachusetts

Francis T. McGovern, M.D.
Instructor in Surgery (Urology)
Harvard Medical School
Division of Urology,
Massachusetts General Hospital,
Boston, Massachusetts

Andrew A. Renshaw, M.D.
Instructor in Pathology,
Harvard Medical School;
Staff Pathologist,
Brigham and Women's Hospital,
Boston, Massachusetts

Jerome P. Richie, M.D.
Elliot Carr Cutler Professor of Urology
Harvard Medical School
Chief, Division of Urology,
Brigham and Women's Hospital,
Boston, Massachusetts

William U. Shipley, M.D., F.A.C.R.
Professor of Radiation Oncology,
Harvard Medical School;
Head, Genitourinary Oncology Unit,
Massachusetts General Hospital,
Boston, Massachusetts

James A. Talcott, M.D., S.M.
Assistant Professor of Medicine,
Harvard Medical School;
Division of Medical Oncology,
Dana-Farber Cancer Institute,
Boston, Massachusetts

Clare M. C. Tempany, M.D.
Assistant Professor of Diagnostic Radiology,
Harvard Medical School;
Director of Body MRI,
Department of Radiology,
Brigham and Women's Hospital,
Boston, Massachusetts

Kenneth I. Wishnow, M.D.
Urology
New England Deaconess Hospital;
Harvard Medical School,
Boston, Massachusetts

Anthony L. Zietman, M.D.
Assistant Professor of Radiation Oncology
Harvard Medical School;
Attending Radiation Oncologist,
Massachusetts General Hospital,
Boston, Massachusetts

Preface

▼ ▼ ▼ ▼ ▼ ▼ ▼ ▼

F EW topics have engendered more controversy in both the medical and lay literature than prostate cancer. Patient and physician alike often come away from reading about prostate cancer more confused and bewildered than when they started.

This book was conceived and designed with several goals in mind. First, we wanted the book to be useful to the interested patient and to physicians who do not routinely care for patients with prostate cancer, as well as to specialists who manage prostate cancer on a daily basis. Second, we wanted the book to be complete but not voluminous. We did not want to produce another textbook on prostate cancer; there are many fine textbooks already available. We wanted a book with chapters that were focused enough to be read in a single sitting. Third, we wanted a balanced view on each topic. Consequently, each chapter has been written by a "team" of coauthors representing different specialties with somewhat different perspectives. Finally, we wanted the reader to receive a critique of the areas of controversy and disagreement. Therefore we have added an editorial comment at the end of each chapter, to try to summarize the crucial issues discussed.

We hope that these efforts have resulted in a book that will be useful to all those interested in the challenge of treating prostate cancer.

Philip W. Kantoff, M.D.
Kenneth I. Wishnow, M.D.
Kevin R. Loughlin, M.D.

Screening for Prostate Cancer: The Horns of a Dilemma

▼ ▼ ▼ ▼ ▼ ▼ ▼ ▼

1

Jerome P. Richie
Irving D. Kaplan

P ROSTATE cancer, the second leading cause of death from cancer among men in the United States, is a major cause of morbidity and mortality. Prostate cancer represents the most common noncutaneous malignancy in men in the United States; in 1996, an estimated 317,100 new cases, and 41,400 deaths, are expected. Based on these statistics, a new patient with prostate cancer will be diagnosed in the United States every 1.7 minutes, and every 13 minutes, one man will die from prostate cancer (1). Traditionally, the digital rectal examination has been used to identify patients with prostate cancer. Unfortunately, however, this test lacks sensitivity and specificity such that most men with prostate cancer detected by digital rectal examination will already have rather extensive disease, making recovery less likely.

In spite of the sobering statistics concerning prostate cancer, there continues to exist considerable debate over the need for early detection and subsequent treatment of prostate cancer.

■ SCREENING

Screening is the use of a test or examination to detect a cancer when no signs or symptoms of the specific cancer are present. Screening for prostate cancer can be defined as a systematic program to identify prostate cancer in a population of asymptomatic men, with subsequent reduction in the mortality rate from this disease. Cancer screening is synonymous with early detection in the general population, although some practitioners will use prostate cancer screening

▼

for patients with an established risk factor, such as strong family history of the disease or African-American background.

Several parameters must be met for screening to be considered effective. First it must be assumed that early treatment, initiated at the time of diagnosis with a screening program, will be more effective than therapy undertaken at a later time (the usual time of diagnosis of the tumor). The disease screened must be considered serious from a health standpoint, and treatments must be efficacious and widely available. Furthermore, testing methods must be safe, relatively inexpensive, rapid, and reproducible, and have acceptable sensitivity, specificity, and positive predictive values.

The gold standard for proof of a screening program is a randomized, controlled trial using cancer-specific mortality as its end point. Such a trial avoids the introduction of potential biases that may result from screening. With certain malignancies, such as breast cancer, screening of asymptomatic persons has been shown to increase survival. With prostate cancer, no randomized prospective trial exists with cancer-specific mortality as an end point to validate screening. To weigh the pros and cons of screening for prostate cancer, a closer look at the pertinent issues and potential biases is warranted.

■ DOES PROSTATE CANCER POSE A SIGNIFICANT HEALTH RISK?

Prostate cancer is now the second leading cause of death in men (1). Furthermore, the incidence of clinically detectable prostate cancer has risen sharply. A 50-year-old man has an approximately 10% risk of developing clinically significant prostate cancer during his lifetime and an overall lifetime risk of 3% of dying from prostate cancer. Prior to the advent of prostate-specific antigen (PSA), more than half of the prostate cancers detected were clinically advanced at the time of diagnosis (2). At the time of diagnosis, distant metastases were noted in approximately 25% of patients. The median survival time for such patients was less than 36 months. Pelvic lymph node metastases were noted in approximately 25% to 30% of patients with clinical organ-confined disease, ranging from 10% to 15% for patients with B1 nodules to greater than 50% for patients with stage C disease.

Adding to the debate over the need for early detection is the fact that prostate cancer is frequently a disease of older men with comorbid disease. Prostate cancer is relatively slow growing as compared to lung or colon cancer. A further confounding factor is the fact that microscopic cancers have been found in up to 50% of older men at the time of autopsy. Thus, many individuals believe that men with prostate cancer will die *with* their disease rather than *from* it. Contributing to an approach of therapeutic nihilism is the fact that many individuals with prostate cancer are incurable at the time of diagnosis.

■ PROSTATE-SPECIFIC ANTIGEN

Several significant factors have added impetus to the issue of screening for prostate cancer. First and foremost was the discovery and subsequent widespread use of PSA, a serine protease, which can be measured in the bloodstream and is elevated in most men with detectable prostate cancer (3). Although this test is associated with false-positive elevations because of benign prostatic hyperplasia, prostatitis, or prostatic infarct, the positive predictive value of PSA is 31%, substantially higher than mammography for the detection of breast cancer. Another factor facilitating diagnosis has been the use of transrectal ultrasonography and spring-loaded biopsy needles to accurately visualize and sample different portions of the prostate with relatively low morbidity or patient discomfort (4). These two factors have resulted in a sharp rise in the diagnosis of prostate cancer from 1986 to 1996. Although many individuals were concerned that clinically unimportant prostate cancers were being detected, with subsequent overtreatment, the American Cancer Society National Prostate Cancer Detection Program, as well as the Hybritech-2 Multi-Institution Screening Center study, have shown that approximately 93% of cancers that are detectable by current methods are clinically important, likely to progress, and of significant volume (5,6). Furthermore, tumors detected by PSA screening have double the likelihood of being organ confined (70%), compared with a 30% to 35% chance for those detected by standard means (5).

■ NATURAL HISTORY

Opponents of screening point to the natural history of prostate cancer as a slow-growing disease and focus on several studies wherein most patients died with prostate cancer but not because of prostate cancer. George, in a series of 120 patients, reported that only 4% of patients died of prostate cancer whereas 40% died of other causes (7). In a widely quoted study of watchful waiting, or conservative management, Johansson and associates followed 233 elderly patients who received treatment only at the time of symptomatic progression (8). Ten percent of their patients died of prostate cancer whereas 84% died of other causes. This study, however, was significantly flawed, as it represented an extremely selected series. Two-thirds of the patients were over 70 years of age and more than one-third of patients has stage A1 prostate cancer. The diagnosis of prostate cancer was made on the basis of transurethral resection of the prostate (TURP). Additionally, in the first two years of the study, only patients with well-differentiated tumors were enrolled, further biasing the results. Progression was determined by bone scan and rectal examination alone. Nonetheless, even in Johansson's series, patients with moderately differentiated disease had a 33% rate of progression, and those with poorly differentiated disease, a 66% rate of progression.

Other studies, however, would contradict the apparent benign nature of prostate cancer described by Johansson. Gronberg and associates examined the records of almost 7,000 men in northern Sweden with detected prostate cancer and compared their survival with that of an age-matched group (9). The relative survival rate of men with prostate cancer was only 45% at 10 years. Furthermore, the decrease in survival was greater in younger men and those with higher grade cancers. Overall, men with prostate cancer lost an average of 40% of their expected longevity. Gann and associates reported in the Physicians Health Study of 22,000 male physicians that 2% developed clinically evident prostate cancer (10). Those cases had a significant excess in mortality, with 75% of the deaths in men with prostate cancer directly attributable to metastatic prostate cancer. In a study at Baylor of 360 men with clinically localized prostate cancer treated with gold seeds and external beam radiation, 54% of the 142 deaths were caused by prostate cancer (11). It would seem, therefore, that prostate cancer is a major cause of death in men who are diagnosed clinically with the disease. Prostate cancer cannot be considered a uniformly benign neoplasm with an indolent course.

Another argument in favor of early detection is the fact that treatment of advanced prostate cancer has not improved substantially since Huggins described hormonal dependence in 1945. The median time to progression after hormonal treatment is 12 to 18 months, and median survival after progression is 12 to 24 months at best (12). By 10 years, three-fourths of men with prostate cancer will die of their disease, for a cancer-specific mortality rate of greater than 90%. Once patients have positive nodal involvement, median time to progression is generally 2 years or less in most series, with virtually all series showing progression by 10 years. Between one-third and one-half of stage D1 patients treated with hormonal ablation will die of their disease within five years. Thus, it seems clear that effective durable treatment is not available for patients in whom prostate cancer has already metastasized.

■ CAN EARLY-STAGE DISEASE BE TREATED EFFECTIVELY?

No prospective randomized study using cancer-specific mortality as its end point has been completed. There are two trials under way. One, sponsored by the National Cancer Institute, is the Prostate, Lung, Colorectal and Ovarian Cancer Screening Trial (PLCO) (13). The Veterans Administration has embarked upon a treatment study called the Prostate (Cancer) Intervention Versus Observation Trial (PIVOT), designed to compare radical prostatectomy with watchful waiting (14). Both of these trials will take many years to accrue patients, with an ultimate long-term follow-up of 10 or 15 years before definitive conclusions can be reached.

Using PSA as a biochemical marker after radical prostatectomy, prognosis for patients can be telescoped from the traditional 10 to 15 years to 5 to 7 years. In patients with organ-confined disease, the likelihood of being free of disease by the most sensitive biochemical (PSA) measurement is 95% at 5 years and 90% at 10 years (15). Thus, it would seem that our goal should be to identify patients with clinically significant prostate cancer at the time that the cancer is organ confined. PSA screening does just that, with more than 90% of patients having clinical evidence of organ-confined disease and 70% of patients having pathologically defined organ-confined disease at the time of radical prostatectomy. This is in contradistinction to the 30% of patients who have organ-confined disease when detected primarily by digital rectal examination. A second important marker for the benefit of early detection is the incidence of positive nodal involvement. Prior to the advent of PSA screening, 25% to 50% of individuals explored were found to have positive pelvic lymph nodes. In the PSA era, the incidence of positive nodes has dropped to 2% to 3% (16). This, too, is likely to translate into long-term disease-free survival.

■ **LEAD TIME AND LENGTH TIME BIAS**

Although it seems logical that earlier detection and treatment of prostate cancer should lead to a decrease in cancer mortality and an overall increase in survival, certain biases must be considered. If screening is to lower the cancer-specific death rate, cancers must be detectable while still curable in men who would otherwise be destined to die of their disease. If early detection simply detects cancers earlier but does not alter progression, these patients would appear to live longer from the time of diagnosis, but overall survival would not be changed. This is called *lead time bias*, the length of time by which screening advances the diagnosis of cancer compared with the standard of clinical detection (17). Thus, if the earlier detection does not alter the natural history of the disease, an apparent increase in survival could be seen without an actual reduction in mortality.

Length time bias occurs when there is biologic variability in the population of cancers (17). Due to the nature of screening programs, cancers with a longer detectable preclinical phase (i.e., slow-growing cancers) are more likely to be detected by screening at various intervals than would those rapidly progressive cancers—those with brief preclinical phases. Individuals with a cancer of the latter type are more likely to die of their disease and less likely to be identified by screening. Therefore, patients with cancers detected by screening who are less likely to have aggressive progression may seem to have a better prognosis than those cancer patients detected in the general population by clinical means, who may have more aggressive tumors.

■ **FINANCIAL IMPLICATIONS**

Perhaps the most problematic of all arguments against widespread early detection or screening for prostate cancer is the potential cost of screening. Such cost would include not only the monetary cost of the screening test but also the costs of subsequent tests performed to validate the initial test—for example, transrectal ultrasound- (TRUS) guided needle biopsies—and subsequent treatment for the cancer. Because of the large number of men in the United States over the age of 50, the cost of early prostate cancer detection and treatment would be measured in billions of dollars. It is unlikely, however, that such an enormous cost would be incurred, as experience generally dictates that only a small percent of patients who are offered screening or early detection will actually participate. In addition, one must factor in the cost of treatment of metastatic disease, albeit with discounted dollars. Watanabe found the total cost for treating advanced prostate cancer to be triple that of treatment of early-stage disease (18). Nonetheless, cost-benefit analysis can be used to analyze the cost of screening and the estimated cost per life saved.

■ APPLICATION OF PSA

In favor of screening is the fact that the American Cancer Society and the American Urological Association have adopted a recommendation to support routine screening for prostate cancer with both digital rectal examination and serum PSA on an annual basis, beginning at age 50. In contrast, however, the U.S. Preventive Services Task Force and the Canadian Task Force on Periodic Health Examination do not recommend routine screening. There is no question that, with application of PSA and de facto screening, substantial numbers of patients with prostate cancer at an earlier stage are being detected, when cure is highly likely. There are two surrogate end points that have been identified by screening studies—the incidence of positive lymph nodes has decreased from 25% to 50% to 2% to 3%, and the incidence of organ-confined disease has increased from 35% to over 70%. In a multicenter screening study of more than 6,000 men, in patients who underwent radical prostatectomy, 93% were found to have *significant disease*, defined as disease involving more than one quadrant of the prostate or moderate or poorly differentiated disease. Thus, although we are identifying significant disease at an earlier stage, without a randomized prospective trial we cannot absolutely prove the efficacy of screening.

To screen or not to screen remains a difficult question. Based on the incidence, prevalence, and identification of significant disease, a strong case can be made for screening men aged 50 to 70 who are otherwise in good health. PSA alone has a positive predictive value of 31%, at least double that of mammography. Importantly, PSA screening should be discouraged for men with a life expectancy of less than 10 years.

Editorial Comment

Few areas in oncology have engendered as much controversy as screening for prostate cancer. As the authors of this chapter point out, the detection of prostate cancer had been inadequate prior to the development of the prostate-specific antigen (PSA) as a screening tool. It appears that, overall, the prostate cancers that have been diagnosed since the introduction and widespread use of the PSA are more likely to be curable, and yet they have the characteristics of cancers that potentially would be of clinical importance. Unfortunately, both of these observations are empirical and the long-term benefits of screening remain uncertain. Were it not for the morbidity of treatment and the cost of treatment, screening for prostate cancer would have widespread support, but until the morbidity of treatment is significantly reduced, we need to continue to look at screening for prostate cancer with some degree of circumspection. Clearly, randomized controlled trials are needed to demonstrate its efficacy. Until such trials are conducted, it seems that the most reasonable approach would be to have the informed patient participate in the decision process. It also seems reasonable to limit screening to populations wherein a benefit might be derived: that is, in men with a life expectancy sufficiently long that the morbidity or mortality of localized prostate cancer may have an impact. A great deal more information regarding screening of high-risk populations, as well as information about which cancers ought to be treated, needs to be obtained before firm recommendations can be made.

■ REFERENCES

1. Parker SL, Tong T, Bolden S, Wingo PA. Cancer statistics, 1996. CA Cancer J Clin 1996;46:5–28.

2. Murphy GP, Natarajan N, Pontes JE, et al. The national survey of prostate cancer in the United States by the American College of Surgeons. J Urol 1982;127:928–934.

3. Catalona WJ, Smith DS, Ratliff TL, et al. Measurement of prostate-specific antigen in serum as a screening test for prostate cancer. N Engl J Med 1994;330:242.

4. Hodge KK, NcNeal JE, Terris MK, Stamey TA. Random systematic versus directed ultrasound guided transrectal core biopsies of the prostate. J Urol 1989;142:71–74.

5. Catalona WJ, Hudson MA, Scardino PT, et al. Selection of optimal prostate-specific antigen cutoffs for early detection of prostate cancer. J Urol 1994;152:2037–2042.

6. Mostofi FK, Murphy GP, Mettlin C, et al. Pathology review in an early prostate cancer detection program: results from the American Cancer Society–National Prostate Cancer Detection Project. Prostate 1995;27:7–12.

7. George NJ. Natural history of localized prostatic cancer managed by conservative therapy alone. Lancet 1988;1:494–497.

8. Johansson JE, Adami HO, Andersson SO, et al. High 10-year survival rate in patients with early, untreated prostatic cancer. JAMA 1992;267:2191.

9. Gronberg H, Damber J, Honsson H, et al. Patient age as a prognostic factor in prostate cancer. J Urol 1994;152:892.

10. Gann PH, Hennekens CH, Stampfer MJ. A prospective evaluation of plasma prostate-specific antigen for detection of prostatic cancer. JAMA 1995;273:28.

11. Lerner SP, Seale HC, Carlton CJ, et al. The risk of dying of prostate cancer in patients with clinically localized disease. J Urol 1991;146:1040.

12. Adolfsson J, Carstensen J, Lowhagen T. Deferred treatment in clinically localized prostatic carcinoma. Br J Urol 1992;69:183.

13. Kramer BS, Gohagan J, Prorok PC, Smart C. A National Cancer Institute–sponsored screening trial for prostatic, lung, colorectal, and ovarian cancers. Cancer 1993;71:589–593.

14. Moon TD, Brawer MK, Wilt TJ. Prostate intervention versus observation trial (PIVOT): a randomized trial comparing radical prostatectomy with palliative expectant management for treatment of clinically localized prostate cancer. NCI Monogr 1995;19:69–71.

15. Walsh PC, Partin AW, Epstein JI. Cancer control and quality of life following anatomical radical retropubic prostatectomy: results at 10 years. J Urol 1994;152:1831–1836.

16. Sullivan LD, Rabbani F. Should we reconsider the indications for ileoobturator node dissection with localized prostate cancer? Br J Urol 1995;75:33–37.

17. Morrison AS. The effects of early treatment, lead time and length time bias on the mortality experienced by cases detected by screening. Int J Epidemiol 1982;11:261–267.

18. Watanabe H. Problems in mass screening program for prostatic diseases. Gan No Rinsho 1984;30:606–610.

Prognostic Features in the Pathology of Prostatic Carcinoma

▼ ▼ ▼ ▼ ▼ ▼ ▼ ▼

2

Andrew A. Renshaw
Christopher L. Corless

PROSTATIC carcinoma is among the most common malignancies of older men and a leading cause of death in this population. Its relatively slow growth and androgen dependence distinguish it from most other carcinomas. Nevertheless, the most important prognostic features of prostatic carcinoma are the same as most other cancers: tumor stage and grade. Over the past three decades the criteria for staging and garding prostatic carcinoma have been refined, allowing reasonably accurate predictions of tumor burden and the chance of tumor progression. Current approaches to the staging and grading of prostatic carcinoma in radical prostatectomy specimens, needle core biopsies, and transurethral resection specimens are reviewed in this chapter. The prognostic utility of prostatic intraepithelial neoplasia (PIN), a putative precursor lesion for prostatic carcinoma, and DNA ploidy analysis are also considered. Finally, new molecular markers are discussed with respect to their potential use in predicting patient prognosis.

■ PROGNOSTIC FEATURES IN RADICAL PROSTATECTOMY SPECIMENS

The typical radical prostatectomy specimen weighs 25 to 75 gm and includes the right and left seminal vesicles and a short segment of the left and right vasa deferentia. Standard pathologic examination begins with the application of ink to the surface of the specimen to mark

▼

the surgical margins, followed by fixation and sectioning of the gland. Although many research-oriented departments prepare entire cross sections of the gland for microscopic examination, most practices rely on selective sampling from both lobes to provide diagnostic material. The accuracy of such selective sampling has been well documented (1–4).

The current standard of practice includes microscopic examination of the periurethral prostatic tissue located at both the apex and base (bladder neck) of the gland—i.e., the distal and proximal resection margins. In addition, the relationship of the tumor to the nearest anterior, lateral, and posterior margins is assessed. Sections of the seminal vesicles are separately examined and reported. Microscopic examination of a tumor allows three parameters to be assessed: grade, stage, and margin status. As discussed below, each of these parameters provides important prognostic information.

Grade

Several grading systems have been developed for prostatic carcinoma, and most have shown correlation with patient survival (5,6). In 1979, a consensus panel reviewed several of these systems and recommended the use of Gleason grading as the standard (5). This system is based entirely on the architectural features of a tumor and ignores cytologic features (7). Architectural patterns are grouped into five grades, numbered 1 through 5, with grade 1 having the best prognosis and grade 5 the worst (Fig. 2.1). Since the majority of tumors have more than one architectural pattern present, the grade of both the predominant architectural pattern as well as the second most common pattern are recorded. The sum of these two grades is the Gleason score, which can range from 2 to 10. Additional Gleason patterns present in a tumor can be commented on in a note, but are not used in the determination of the Gleason score.

In part because of its simplicity, the Gleason grading scheme provides good interobserver reproducibility (5,8,9). In one study, agreement among pathologists when measured against consensus scores was 74% to 93%, although variation from the consensus score by one Gleason point was allowed (10). Exact agreement between

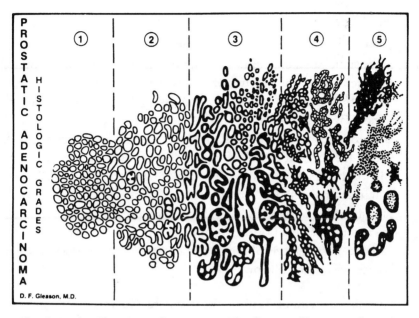

Fig. 2.1 *The Gleason grading system. The diagram illustrates the architectural pattern of the neoplastic glands. (Reproduced by permission of Dr. D. F. Gleason.)*

pathologists is only about 50% (9,10). Intraobserver reproducibility using the Gleason grading scheme is also good (10).

Gleason scores clearly correlate with patient survival and have a prognostic impact independent of tumor stage (7,11–17). Low-grade tumors (Gleason score of 2 to 4) have an excellent prognosis but unfortunately make up a small minority of all resected cancers. The majority of patients have tumors with Gleason scores in the intermediate range (5 to 7). Prognosis for this group is significantly better than that for patients with high-grade tumors (scores 8 to 10). However, the prognosis of patients with intermediate-grade tumors is quite variable.

Recent studies suggest that patients with Gleason score 7 tumors have a significantly worse prognosis than patients with Gleason score 5 or 6 tumors (15,18). This may be related to a high rate of extraprostatic spread among tumors with a high Gleason score; organ-confined tumors of Gleason score 7 or higher may have a very good prognosis (18).

Stage

The stage of a tumor is the single most important prognostic factor in prostatic carcinoma (6,15). When properly examined and sampled for microscopy, the staging of radical prostatectomy specimens is straightforward. All information necessary to establish pathologic tumor stage using the tumor-nodes-metastasis (TNM) system (which is more precise than the Marshall-Jewett system) should be included within the surgical pathology report. The relative volume and laterality of the tumor should be given, and the relationship to all resection margins detailed. Unfortunately, standardized reporting of prostatectomy specimens has only recently been promoted (19), and the amount of detail provided in pathology reports remains highly variable. Basic aspects of tumor and node staging for prostatic carcinomas are outlined below.

Location of Tumor Within the Prostate Gland: Three anatomic zones have been defined for the prostate gland: transitional (periurethral), central (around the ejaculatory ducts), and peripheral (a horseshoe-shaped area enveloping the posterior and lateral aspects of the gland). Approximately 80% of carcinomas arise in the peripheral zone (20–22). Overall, transition zone tumors tend to be smaller in volume and lower in grade than peripheral zone tumors (22), and they are less likely to exhibit DNA aneuploidy (23); all these features portend a better prognosis. Among tumors of like grade, however, it is unclear whether the zone of origin influences prognosis. Moreover, most prostatic carcinomas are multifocal (20), so assigning a site of origin is often difficult.

Tumor Volume: More important than zonal origin is an estimation of the tumor volume. Small, nodular tumors that occupy less than half of one lobe (stage T2a) are more likely to be organ-confined and therefore carry a better prognosis than tumors that occupy more than half of a lobe (stage T2b) or are bilateral (stage T2c). Unfortunately, bilateral glandular involvement is the most common finding in prostatectomy specimens.

Whether estimation of tumor volume provides prognostic information that is independent of Gleason score remains an unsettled question. It is well documented that very large tumors (e.g., greater than 12 cc in volume) have a high rate of metastasis, while small tumors (<0.5 cc) metastasize much less often (20,24,25). On the other hand, larger tumors often have higher Gleason scores (26). While some authors feel tumor volume is prognostically significant independent of other parameters (24,25,27), agreement on this point is not universal (14,28,29). Finally, accurate assessment of tumor volume is technically demanding and labor intensive. Thus, while methods for quantitative tumor volume assessment on routinely processed tissue are available (3,4,30), most practicing pathologists report only estimates of the relative amount of tumor within the gland.

Invasion of Tumor Outside the Prostate Gland and the Myth of the Prostate "Capsule": One of the more controversial aspects of prostatic carcinoma staging is determining whether a tumor has left the confines of the gland and invaded extraprostatic tissues. This is in part due to a long-standing perpetuation of the myth that the prostate gland has a capsule. Unlike kidney, liver, and spleen, the prostate does not have a well-delineated fibrous capsule surrounding its surface; rather, it is enveloped by a variably condensed band of fibromuscular tissue that arises from the prostatic stroma and separates the glands from adjacent skeletal muscle, fat, and neurovascular connective tissue (31). Since the majority of tumors arise in the peripheral region (20–22), many are found near or within the outermost fibrous strands of the gland. Pathologists must then evaluate whether a tumor invades into or through this poorly defined "capsule," thus distinguishing between a stage T2 tumor that approaches the outer limits of the prostate gland, and a stage T3 tumor that extends beyond the prostate. Tumors with invasion into but not through the outer band of fibromuscular tissue have the same prognosis as those without "capsular" invasion (20). Therefore, so long as the natural contour of the gland is intact and there is no significant stromal desmoplasia, tumor present within the outermost fibrous layers should be interpreted conservatively. However, in some cases this interpretation may be difficult, and differences of opinion may exist.

The significance of extraprostatic spread of tumor is unequivocal; higher rates of recurrence (15,32) and metastasis (13,18) result in decreased overall survival (32) compared with patients who have

organ-confined tumors. Nevertheless, the presence of capsular penetration is not as significant as lymph node or seminal vesicle involvement (13,15,25,32–34). Moreover, the extent of tumor outside the
prostate appears to influence prognosis; there is less chance of disease progression if only focal, as opposed to extensive, extraprostatic
invasion is identified (15,35). Whether the negative prognostic impact
of extraprostatic spread is mitigated by complete resection of the
tumor (negative margins) is less clear (15).

Invasion of the Seminal Vesicles: Stage T3c is defined as invasion of
one or both seminal vesicles by tumor. Several studies have documented that seminal vesicle involvement is a grave prognostic factor
(13,15,20,32–34,36), correlating with positive lymph nodes in up to
50% of cases. The significance of seminal vesicle involvement may
depend in part on the pattern of tumor invasion. Thus, direct invasion into the muscularis of the seminal vesicle may connote a worse
prognosis than the presence of tumor within soft tissues adjacent
to the seminal vesicle (37). More studies are needed to sort out
the relative significance of the various patterns of seminal vesicle
involvement.

Lymph Nodes: The identification of lymph node metastases is generally straightforward. However, it is well documented that the use
of frozen sections to examine grossly normal lymph nodes at the time
of radical prostatectomy is associated with a small false-negative rate
(3.5% of all patients, 27.5% of all patients with positive nodes), which
is presumably due to sampling (38). There is some evidence that the
extent of metastatic tumor may influence survival (39). However, the
presence of any lymph node metastases is a very poor prognostic
sign (15).

Margins

Due to the close anatomic relationship of the prostate with its surrounding structures, including bladder and rectum, there is relatively little soft tissue that can be excised with the prostate to ensure
negative margins. This is reflected in the high overall rate of positive
margins (nearly 40%) reported in many series of retropubic radical

prostatectomies (40). The majority of these margins are near the apex, where there is the least amount of soft tissue surrounding the prostate, and in the posterolateral areas where the tumors tend to arise (40). However, one large series of specimens obtained from a perineal approach documented a high rate of positive anterior margins (41). Thus, the surgical approach may also influence margin status.

The interpretation of surgical margins is complicated by several procedural issues. First, the chance of finding a positive margin is influenced by the amount of sampling (1,2,42). For this reason, most if not all margin tissue present near a grossly identified tumor nodule should be submitted and examined microscopically. Second, the use of en face (shave) sections to evaluate the apical and bladder resection margins leads to a higher frequency of apparent positivity, because even the thinnest of such sections may contain tumor that is not truly at the ink. This approach, which has been abandoned by many pathologists, should be kept in mind when evaluating the significance of a positive apical or bladder margin. Finally, the significance of posterolateral margins is influenced by whether the surgical plane of dissection yields a smooth, natural contour or a ragged, partially incised profile. When tumor is directly adjacent to the inked margin, the probability of inadequate resection appears to be lower for specimens with smooth contours than for those with ragged edges (43).

Since the identification of positive resection margins may influence decisions about postoperative radiation treatments, there should be close communication between pathologists and clinicians concerning the extent of tumor being interpreted as "at the margin." With this in mind, the presence of positive margins is clearly associated with disease progression (15).

■ **PROGNOSTIC FEATURES IN NEEDLE BIOPSIES**

In the United States, needle core biopsies are the favored method for obtaining diagnostic material from the prostate gland. In Europe, fine needle aspiration biopsy (FNA) remains popular. While FNA is both sensitive and specific for the diagnosis of carcinoma (44,45), it has several limitations. First, Gleason grading cannot be done, although cytologic grading is possible. Second, tumor volume, perineural invasion, and extension into fibroadipose tissue, all of which may be prognostically important, cannot be assessed (46). Because of this, FNA is most useful for the diagnosis of recurrent or metastatic disease rather than for initial diagnosis.

For core needle biopsies, several features have been found to be of prognostic importance, including Gleason score, extent of tumor, perineural invasion, extension into fibroadipose tissue, the presence of PIN, and DNA ploidy.

Grade

Despite the limited sample provided by needle biopsy, the correlation between Gleason score on needle biopsy and the subsequent prostatectomy is good. With 14-gauge needles, the assigned Gleason score was within one point of the prostatectomy score 59% to 74% of the time (47,48). Similar studies with 18-gauge needles have shown the same correlation between 74% and 94% of the time (49–51). In all of these studies there is a trend to undergrade rather than overgrade a tumor on needle biopsy; however, this trend does not correlate with clinical understaging.

Extent of Tumor

In general, there is a strong correlation between the amount of tumor seen in a needle biopsy and the amount found at radical prostatectomy (52,53). Nevertheless, extensive tumor has been found in prostatectomy specimens after biopsies showed only minimal tumor involvement (54–56).

Using various combinations of clinical and pathologic parameters it is possible to assign a relative probability that a given tumor is of "clinically significant" volume—that is, greater than 0.2 cc (53,56) or 0.5 cc (52,57). Perhaps half of all patients with normal serum PSA or PSA density and small amounts of well to moderately differentiated tumor (Gleason score <7) on biopsy will have a tumor under 0.2 to 0.5 cc in volume at prostatectomy (52,53,56,57). Nevertheless, for the individual patient it is currently not possible to make preoperative determinations of either the volume or stage of prostate cancer with 100% accuracy (51).

Perineural Invasion

In one large study, the presence of perineural invasion in a needle biopsy was a specific although insensitive marker for extracapsular extension (58). This observation may reflect a tumor's tendency to invade extraprostatic tissue by way of perineural spaces (59).

Extension into Nonprostatic Tissue

The presence of prostatic carcinoma in adipose tissue is highly suggestive of extracapsular spread. The presence of prostatic carcinoma in association with ganglion cells is also suggestive, but not diagnostic, of extracapsular spread (60).

Prostatic Intraepithelial Neoplasia

As detailed below, PIN is currently viewed as a premalignant precursor of invasive carcinoma. Its identification on needle biopsy is a strong indication for rebiopsy. Between 50% and 100% of men with PIN will demonstrate carcinoma on a concurrent or subsequent biopsy (61–63).

■ **PROGNOSTIC FEATURES IN TRANSURETHRAL RESECTION SPECIMENS**

Transurethral resections (TURs) are performed for obstructive symptoms. Prostatic carcinomas detected in the "chips" are either incidental or else recurrent lesions that may be the cause of the obstruction. Incidental prostatic carcinomas are the focus of further consideration.

Most of the tissue removed by TUR is from the periurethral area, corresponding to the central and transitional zones of the prostate. Carcinomas found in this region are often smaller and of a lower grade than those found in the peripheral zone (22). Incidental carcinomas are found in about 10% to 15% of TUR specimens done for prostatic hypertrophy. By definition these tumors are stage A (Whitmore-Jewett system) or T1 (TMN system). In 1981, a group from Johns Hopkins University segregated stage A1 tumors (Gleason score <5 or involvement of less than 5% of the resected tissue) from A2 tumors (Gleason score 5 or more and greater than 5% of the resected tissue) and assessed the relative risk of progression in a group of untreated patients (64). Stage A2 patients had a significantly higher risk of progression (32%) over a four-year period than those with stage A1 (2%). In studies with a longer follow-up time, the rate of progression in stage A1 patients is higher: 10% at 7 years, 16% at 8 years, and 25% at 10.2 years (65–67). These observations correlate well with a recent analysis of 64 prostatectomy specimens resected for TUR-detected stage A1 cancer, in which 20% of the cases contained substantial residual tumor (68). Stage A2 patients are thought to be candidates for further treatment, either by surgical resection or radiotherapy (69). In view of the increasing progression rate with longer follow-up, younger patients with stage A1 disease may also be candidates for treatment.

The difference in prognosis between stage A1 and A2 has stimulated much debate on how best to measure the percent of tissue involved by tumor. Some experts prefer to make visual estimates of the percentage area of chips containing tumor (64,70,71), while others prefer a ratio of chips involved to total number of chips (72,73). The introduction of the TNM staging system defines stage T1a as having three or fewer microscopic foci and T1b as more than three microscopic foci. Gleason score is not included in the TNM system.

Regardless of the classification system used, the amount of tumor identified in TUR specimens is dependent on the number of chips examined microscopically (74,75). Ideally all tissue should be examined, but in large samples this becomes impractical. Some authors suggest that sampling of up to 12 gm of chips will detect up to 90% of T1a tumors and all T1b tumors (76,77). Similarly, all stage A2 cancers can probably be detected by submitting enough chips to fill five to eight paraffin blocks (78,79). However, others feel that 95% of the tissue must be examined to detect 95% of all tumors (80). Currently the College of American Pathologists recommends submitting at least 12 gm of tissue, and if a stage T1a cancer is found, submission of the remaining tissue (19).

■ PROSTATIC INTRAEPITHELIAL NEOPLASIA

Descriptions of putative precursor lesions of prostatic carcinoma date back at least to 1965 (8,81). The entities and terms include atypical hyperplasia (82,83), intraductal carcinoma (84), atypical foci (85), and, most recently, prostatic intraepithelial neoplasia (86). Originally PIN was defined by three grades, but a simpler two-tier system of high and low grade has since been adopted (87). The evidence linking PIN with carcinoma is much stronger for high-grade than low-grade PIN; consequently, for the remainder of this section, only high-grade PIN will be discussed.

The evidence linking PIN with carcinoma is both circumstantial and morphologic. The evidence that PIN is spatially associated with carcinoma is overwhelming (86,88–92). The nuclear morphology of PIN is similar to prostatic carcinoma (93,94). In addition, the DNA ploidy of PIN often matches that of any coexistent carcinoma (95–98).

However, direct demonstration of PIN progressing to carcinoma is not possible, because the lesions are microscopic and cannot be both biopsied and observed. In an epidemiologic approach to this problem, autopsy prostates from men with no history of prostate cancer were examined for the presence of PIN, incidental carcinoma, or both. Surprisingly, PIN was not more common than invasive carcinoma in this population, nor did PIN appear in men younger than those with carcinoma (99). One explanation for these findings might be that PIN lesions are rapidly overrun by an evolving tumor and are therefore no longer recognizable. Nevertheless, it is also possible that many lesions of PIN simply represent intraductal spread of an otherwise invasive carcinoma.

What, then, is the significance of PIN in specimens of prostate tissue? As reviewed above, in needle biopsies PIN is a strong predictor of coexistent invasive carcinoma, and may indicate the need for further biopsies if carcinoma is not identified in the concurrent biopsy.

■ VARIANTS OF PROSTATIC CARCINOMA

Large Duct (Endometrioid) Carcinoma

Large duct carcinoma of the prostate was originally termed endometrioid carcinoma because it was thought to arise from müllerian remnants found in the prostatic utricle (100). Several series have since documented that this type of carcinoma originates from the large, periurethral ducts of the prostate and is both prostate-specific antigen (PSA) and prostatic acid phosphatase (PAP) immunoreactive (101–104). Histologically, the tumor is distinguished by tall columnar cells arranged in papillary configurations and is quite different from the typical acinar pattern of prostatic carcinoma. In most cases, however, large duct carcinoma is not pure but is instead associated with typical carcinoma. Large duct carcinoma is uncommon, and it appears to be more aggressive than typical carcinoma, although many of the cases in these series were high stage and unresected.

Mucinous Adenocarcinoma of the Prostate

Focal mucin positivity is relatively common in typical prostatic adenocarcinoma, reported in up to 33% of cases (105). Mucinous carcinomas, defined as having "lakes" of mucin occupying at least 25% of the tumor volume (106), are quite rare (0.4% of cases). Because of sampling issues, mucinous tumors cannot be definitively identified by needle biopsy. The tumor cells associated with the mucin lakes are usually intermediate grade; however, the nonmucinous portions of the tumor are often high grade (106,107). The tumor cells are immunoreactive for PSA and PAP. Significantly, signet ring cells are not present. The prognosis is uncertain, due to the small number of cases that have been studied. There is controversy as to whether these tumors are sensitive to estrogen.

Signet-Ring Cell Prostatic Carcinoma

Signet-ring cell carcinoma of the prostate is an extremely uncommon tumor. There are case reports of mucin-positive, PSA- and PAP-negative tumors, but the origin of these tumors is uncertain (108). In contrast, one study documented cases of signet-ring cell carcinoma that were mucin negative and PSA and PAP positive (109). These tumors probably represent variants of very poorly differentiated prostatic carcinoma (Gleason score 9 or 10). All were unresectable, advanced tumors with a poor prognosis (108, 109).

Neuroendocrine Differentiation in Prostatic Carcinoma and Small Cell Carcinoma

Cells exhibiting neuroendocrine differentiation are normal constituents of the adult prostate gland (110). Between 47% and 100% of prostatic carcinomas have at least focal neuroendocrine differentiation when examined using immunohistochemical techniques (111–116). Neuroendocrine cells can also be detected in metastatic tumor deposits (117,118). Several studies have assigned prognostic value to the finding of neuroendocrine differentiation in prostate tumors (114–116,119), but it is found with such high frequency that its effect may be diluted beyond significance.

Neuroendocrine differentiation is also characteristic of small cell carcinoma of the prostate. However, the diagnosis of small cell carcinoma is made on routine hematoxylin-eosinstained slides. In other words, small cell carcinoma is a histologic diagnosis, not an immunohistochemical diagnosis. However, immunohistochemical staining for neuroendocrine markers can be confirmatory in cases in which small cell carcinoma is suspected. Unlike typical carcinomas with focal neuroendocrine differentiation, small cell carcinomas of the prostate are histologically undifferentiated, most closely resembling oat cell carcinoma of the lung. These tumors are generally negative for PSA and PAP, but may stain positively for chromogranin, synaptophysin, or neuron-specific enolase (120,121). Approximately 40% of small cell carcinomas of the prostate develop months to years after a diagnosis of well to moderately differentiated carcinoma is established (120–124). The remainder present as rapidly evolving cancers that may be either histologically pure small cell carcinoma or intermixed with typical carcinoma. Regardless of the setting in which they arise, small cell carcinomas behave as hormonally independent tumors and are uniformly associated with a poor prognosis; reported median survivals range from 5 to 17 months. Response to chemotherapy has been reported in a few cases, but a survival benefit has not been demonstrated (124–126).

Basal Cell Hyperplasia, Basal Cell Tumor, Adenoid Cystic Tumor

Basal cell lesions span a spectrum from focal hyperplasia to well-circumscribed nodules to infiltrative masses. Most often these lesions are found in transurethral resection specimens for prostatic hypertrophy (127). Histologically they show peripheral palisading, squamous metaplasia, and luminal mucin or basement membrane–like material. Occasionally cases resemble adenoid cystic carcinoma of other sites.

The proliferating basal cells are PSA and PAP negative, and instead react for high molecular weight keratins (34βE12) (128,129). Case reports of this tumor abound (130–138), and several small series have been reported (127–129,139). Only one example of extraprostatic extension has been documented (137); no cases of metastasis or death have been attributed to this lesion.

Sarcomatoid Carcinoma

Prostatic carcinomas that show areas of sarcomatous transformation are rare. Based on two small series (140,141), such tumors either present as primary carcinosarcoma of the prostate, or else evolve from an adenocarcinoma after treatment with radiation. The sarcomatous areas exhibit variable residual epithelial differentiation when examined by immunohistochemistry and electron microscopy. Heterologous elements (cartilage, bone) have been identified in some cases. Survival is poor, with a mean time to death of only 12 months (142,143).

■ DNA PLOIDY

DNA ploidy in prostatic carcinoma has been examined in a number of recent studies according to several different approaches. Interpretation of these studies is complicated by three factors. First, there are several methods for determining DNA ploidy, including flow cytometric analysis of nuclei prepared from either fresh tissue or paraffin-embedded tissue, and static image analysis of Feulgen-stained sections. Each of these approaches has technical limitations and may be subject to difficulties in interpretation (144–147). Second, all possible types of specimens across all pathologic stages have been examined in these studies, so that comparisons between them must be made with care. Third, most prostatic carcinomas are multifocal (20), and DNA ploidy can vary among different foci of the same tumor (148). Thus, sampling is crucial in assessing DNA ploidy in prostatic carcinoma.

With the above factors in mind, certain trends with respect to DNA ploidy in prostatic carcinoma can be identified. First, there is a clear correlation between DNA aneuploidy and both higher Gleason score and higher tumor stage (149–154). So while DNA ploidy is correlated with survival (142,155), at issue is whether the detection of an aneuploid cell population within a prostate cancer is prognostically significant independent of Gleason score and stage. For patients who do not go on to radical prostatectomy, DNA ploidy on needle biopsy may provide additional prognostic information in lieu of pathologic staging (143,156–158). In a case-matched control study of biopsies from clinically localized tumors treated with radiation, DNA aneuploidy proved to be an independent predictor of survival (159). In tumors detected in TUR chips, aneuploidy may be a significant predictor for disease progression (160), but its role in predicting survival is uncertain (143,161,162). Finally, in radical prostatectomy specimens there are conflicting data. In some studies, aneuploidy is an independent predictor of either disease progression or survival, or both (162–166), but other studies fail to confirm these observations (146,167,168). Thus, the role of DNA ploidy analysis in radical prostatectomy specimens remains unsettled.

■ MOLECULAR BIOLOGY OF PROSTATIC CARCINOMA

A variety of molecular genetic techniques have recently been applied to the study of prostatic carcinomas, including karyotyping, loss-of-heterozygosity analysis, comparative genomic hybridization, and direct gene sequencing (169–172). Several chromosomal abnormalities have consistently been documented in prostate tumors, particularly deletions in chromosomes 7, 8, 10, 16, 17, and 18. Efforts to identify possible tumor suppressor genes at these loci are well under way. As new genes, such as the prostate cancer metastasis suppressor gene KAI1, are identified specific molecular biological tests will become available to detect their alteration (173).

One tumor suppressor gene that has already received attention as a possible prognostic factor in prostatic carcinoma is p53. The most commonly altered gene in human cancers, p53 plays central roles in both cell cycle control and the regulation of apoptosis (174). Specific assays have been developed to detect mutations and deletions in the p53 gene, and overexpression of the p53 protein (which is commonly the result of mutations) can be measured immunohistochemically. Each of these approaches has recently been applied to prostatic carcinomas (172), and it appears that the gene is commonly altered only in very advanced tumors (175–177). Altered p53 is detected in only 2.7% to 11% of clinically localized tumors (178–182), but it can be found in 15% to 66% of locally invasive and metastatic lesions (177–183). When applied to specific subgroups of patients, particularly those with tumors that have a Gleason score of 2 to 7, p53 may provide additional prognostic information (184).

Cellular oncogenes have also received attention as potential prognostic indicators in prostatic carcinoma. To date, studies of c-erbB-2 (HER-2/neu) (185,186) and ras (187) do not support their use in the routine evaluation of prostate tumors, but many other genes have yet to be examined. The recent identification of mutations in the androgen receptor gene of hormonally independent prostate cancers may be a harbinger of a coming era of molecular pathology (188). It is possible that testing for mutations in a combination of tumor suppressor genes, cellular oncogenes, and adhesion molecules may ultimately prove of greater prognostic importance than tumor grade or stage.

■ CONCLUSION

Over the past three decades, the grading and staging of prostatic carcinoma has been refined and is now applied by pathologists with good reproducibility. When combined with radiologic imaging studies and serum PSA, the pathologic features of prostatic carcinoma are of significant prognostic value and may influence the choice of therapeutic options. It is clear that patients who have small tumors with a low Gleason score have an excellent prognosis and, conversely, that patients with larger, poorly differentiated carcinomas often suffer progression of their disease. Unfortunately, the majority of patients, including those with PSA-detected tumors, have carcinomas that are intermediate in grade and stage, for which the prognosis is quite variable. Future refinements in the staging of resected prostate carcinoma may provide additional prognostic information; however, it is unlikely that the microscope alone will yield what every clinician and patient wants to know: the definitive prognosis for an individual cancer. Such information necessarily lies within the genetic alterations of an evolving carcinoma, and it is here that the frontier of molecular pathology is being established. In the meantime, our current understanding of prostate pathology can best serve the needs of patients through good communication between pathologists and clinicians. A recent trend toward the standardization of surgical pathology reports may help reduce problems in their interpretation, but familiarity with the procedures and terminology used by the local pathology laboratory is still the best course.

Editorial Comment

The reader should recognize that the pathologic characteristics of the primary tumor have a major impact on disease progression and ultimate curability. The Gleason score (range 2 to 10) is one of the major prognostic indicators of tumor behavior. Although not every pathology department uses the Gleason scoring system, it is becoming very widely accepted. As the authors mention, the Gleason score on a needle biopsy generally correlates well with the Gleason score of the surgical specimen.

The significance of positive surgical margins is also reviewed by the authors. It is important to remember that the positive margin rate is influenced somewhat by the preparation of the tissue and the experience of the pathologist.

The presence of prostatic intraepithelial neoplasia (PIN) on needle biopsy needs to be interpreted in the proper context. Detection of high-grade PIN in a needle biopsy specimen is a strong predictor of associated invasive carcinoma, and the patient should be rebiopsied. Whether to rebiopsy patients found to have low-grade PIN on needle biopsy is more problematic. That decision should be influenced by the patient's age, serum PSA, rectal exam, and clinical suspicion.

Although DNA ploidy has been reported to be a useful predictor of the clinical behavior of prostate cancer, it is still more of a research tool than a practical clinical marker. At present, DNA ploidy determinations are not part of the routine pathologic evaluation of prostate cancer specimens in most hospitals.

■ **REFERENCES**

1. Humphrey PA. Complete histologic serial sectioning of a prostate gland with adenocarcinoma. Am J Surg Pathol 1993;17:468–472.

2. Cohen MB, Soloway MS, Murphy WM. Sampling of radical prostatectomy specimens: how much is adequate? Am J Clin Pathol 1994;101:250–252.

3. Hall GS, Kramer CE, Epstein JI. Evaluation of radical prostatectomy specimens: a comparative analysis of sampling methods. Am J Surg Pathol 1992;16:315–324.

4. Schmid HP, McNeal JE. An abbreviated standard procedure for accurate tumor volume estimation in prostate cancer. Am J Surg Pathol 1992;16:184–191.

5. Murphy GP, Whitmore WF. A report of the workshop on the current status of the histologic grading of prostatic cancer. Cancer 1979;44: 1490–1494.

6. Jewett J. Radical perineal prostatectomy for palpable, clinically localized, nonobstructive cancer: experience at The Johns Hopkins Hospital 1909–1963. J Urol 1980;124:492–494.

7. Gleason DF, Mellinger GT. Prediction of prognosis for prostatic adenocarcinoma by combined histologic grading and clinical stage. J Urol 1974;111:58–64.

8. Gleason DF. Atypical hyperplasia, benign hyperplasia, and well-differentiated adenocarcinoma of the prostate. Am J Surg Pathol 1985; 9S:53–67.

9. Gleason DF. Histologic grading of prostate cancer: a perspective. Hum Pathol 1992;23:273–279.

10. Bain GO, Koch M, Hanson J. Feasibility of grading prostatic carcinomas. Arch Pathol Lab Med 1982;106:265–267.

11. Kramer SA, Spahr J, Brendler CB, et al. Experience with Gleason's histopathologic grading in prostatic cancer. J Urol 1980;124:223–224.

12. Sogani PC, Israel A, Lieberman PH, et al. Gleason grading of prostate cancer: a predictor of survival. Urology 1985;25:223–227.

13. Fowler JE, Mills SE. Operable prostatic carcinoma: correlations among clinical stage, pathological stage, Gleason histologic score and early disease-free survival. J Urol 1985;134:49–52.

14. Partin AW, Epstein JI, Cho KR, et al. Morphometric measurement of tumor volume and percent of gland involvement as predictors of pathological stage in clinical stage B prostate cancer. J Urol 1989; 141:341–345.

15. Epstein JI, Pizov G, Walsh PC. Correlation of pathologic findings with progression after radical retropubic prostatectomy. Cancer 1993;71: 3582–3593.

16. Zagars GK, von Eschenbach AC, Ayala AG. Prognostic factors in prostate cancer: analysis of 874 patients treated with radiation therapy. Cancer 1993;72:1709–1725.

17. Sgrignoli AR, Walsh PC, Weinberg GD, et al. Prognostic factors in men with stage D1 prostate cancer: identification of patients less likely to have prolonged survival after radical prostatectomy. J Urol 1994; 152:1077–1081.

18. Ohori M, Goad JR, Wheeler TM, et al. Can radical prostatectomy alter the progression of poorly differentiated prostate cancer? J Urol 1994; 152:1843–1849.

19. Henson DE, Hutter RVP, Farrow G. Practice protocol for the examination of specimens removed from patients with carcinoma of the prostate gland. Arch Pathol Lab Med 1994;118:779–783.

20. Byar DP, Mostofi FK. Carcinoma of the prostate: prognostic evaluation of certain pathologic features in 208 radical prostatectomies. Cancer 1972;30:5–13.

21. McNeal JE. Regional morpholoy and pathology of the prostate. Am J Clin Pathol 1968;49:347–357.

22. McNeal JE, Redwine EA, Freiha FS, Stamey TA. Zonal distribution of prostatic adenocarcinoma. Am J Surg Pathol 1988;12:897–906.

23. Greene DR, Rogers E, Wessels EC, et al. Some small prostate cancers are nondiploid by nuclear image analysis: correlation of deoxyribonucleic acid ploidy status and pathologic features. J Urol 1994;151: 1301–1307.

24. Stamey TA, McNeal JE, Freiha FS, Redwine E. Morphometric and clinical studies on 68 consecutive radical prostatectomies. J Urol 1988;139:1235–1241.

25. McNeal JE, Villers AA, Redwine EA, et al. Capsular penetration in prostate cancer: significance for natural history and treatment. Am J Surg Pathol 1990;14:240–247.

26. McNeal JE, Villers AA, Redwine EA, et al. Histologic differentiation, cancer volume, and pelvic lymph node metastases in adenocarcinoma of the prostate. Cancer 1990;66:1225–1233.

27. Humphrey PA, Frazier HA, Vollmer RT, Paulson DF. Stratification of pathologic features in radical prostatectomy specimens that are predictive of elevated initial postoperative serum prostate-specific antigen levels. Cancer 1993;71:1821–1827.

28. Epstein JI. The prostate and seminal vesicles. In: Sternberg SS, ed. Diagnostic surgical pathology. Vol. 2. New York: Raven Press, 1994:1807–1854.

29. Epstein JI, Carmichael M, Partin AW, Walsh PC. Is tumor volume an independent predictor of progression following radical prostatectomy? A multivariate analysis of 185 clinical stage B adenocarcinomas of the prostate with 5 years of followup. J Urol 1993;149:1478–1481.

30. Humphrey PA, Vollmer RT. Intraglandular tumor extent and prognosis in prostate carcinoma. Hum Pathol 1990;21:799–804.

31. Ayala AG, Ro JY, Babaian R, et al. The prostatic capsule: does it exist? Its importance in the staging and treatment of prostatic carcinoma. Am J Surg Pathol 1989;13:21–27.

32. Stein A, DeKernion JB, Smith RB, et al. Prostate specific antigen levels after radical prostatectomy in patients with organ confined and locally extensive prostate cancer. J Urol 1992;147:942–946.

33. Middleton RG, Smith JA, Melzer RB, Hamilton PE. Patient survival and local recurrence rate following radical prostatectomy for prostatic carcinoma. J Urol 1986;136:422–424.

34. Schellhammer PF. Radical prostatectomy: patterns of local failure and survival in 67 patients. Urology 1988;31:191–197.

35. Epstein JI, Carmichael MJ, Pizov G, Walsh PC. Influence of capsular penetration on progression following radical prostatectomy: a study of 196 cases with long-term followup. J Urol 1993;150:135–141.

36. Jewett HJ. The results of radical perineal prostatectomy. JAMA 1969;210:324–325.

37. Epstein JI, Carmichael M, Walsh PC. Adenocarcinoma of the prostate invading the seminal vesicle: definition and relation of tumor volume, grade and margins of resection to prognosis. J Urol 1993;149: 1040–1045.

38. Epstein JI, Oesterling JE, Eggelston JC, Walsh PC. Frozen section detection of lymph node metastases in prostatic carcinoma: accuracy in grossly uninvolved pelvic lymphadenectomy specimens. J Urol 1986;136:1234–1237.

39. Smith JA, Middleton RG. Implications of volume of nodal metastasis in patients with adenocarcinoma of the prostate. J Urol 1985;133: 617–619.

40. Ackerman DA, Barry JM, Wicklund RA, et al. Analysis of risk factors associated with prostate cancer extension to the surgical margin and pelvic lymph node metastasis at radical prostatectomy. J Urol 1993;150:1845–1850.

41. Weldon VE, Tavel FR, Neuwirth H, Cohen R. Patterns of positive specimen margins and detectable prostate specific antigen after radical perineal prostatectomy. J Urol 1995;153:1565–1569.

42. Haggman M, Norberg M, de la Torre M, et al. Characterization of localized prostatic cancer: distribution, grading and pT staging in radical prostatectomy specimens. Scand J Urol Nephrol 1993;27: 7–13.

43. Epstein JI. Evaluation of radical prostatectomy capsular margins of resection: the significance of margins designated negative, closely approaching and positive. Am J Surg Pathol 1990;14:626–632.

44. Lijung BM, Cherrie R, Kaufman JJ. Fine needle aspiration biopsy of the prostate gland: a study of 103 cases with histologic follow-up. J Urol 1986;135:955–958.

45. Ritchie AWS, Layfield LJ, Turcillo P, de Kernion JB. The significance of atypia in fine needle aspiration cytology of the prostate. J Urol 1988;140:761–765.

46. Eble JN, Angermeier PA. The role of fine needle aspiration and needle core biopsies in the diagnosis of primary prostatic cancer. Hum Pathol 1992;23:249–257.

47. Catalona WJ, Stein AJ, Fair WR. Grading errors in prostatic needle biopsies: relation to the accuracy of tumor grade in predicting pelvic lymph node metastases. J Urol 1982;127:919–922.

48. Mills SE, Fowler JE. Gleason histologic grading of prostatic carcinoma: correlations between biopsy and prostatectomy specimens. Cancer 1986;57:346–349.

49. Spires SE, Cibull ML, Wood DP, et al. Gleason histologic grading in prostatic carcinoma. Correlation of 18 gauge core biopsy with prostatectomy. Arch Pathol Lab Med 1994;118:705–708.

50. Bostwick DG. Gleason grading of prostatic needle biopsies. Correlation with grade in 316 matched prostatectomies. Am J Surg Pathol 1994;18:796–803.

51. Humphrey PA, Baty J, Keetch D. Relationship between serum prostate specific antigen, needle biopsy findings, and histopathologic features of prostatic carcinoma in radical prostatectomy tissues. Cancer 1995;75:1842–1849.

52. Goto Y, Ohori M, Arakawa A, et al. Distinguishing clinically important from unimportant prostate cancers before treatment: preliminary report. J Urol 1994;151(suppl):289A. Abstract.

53. Epstein JI, Walsh PC, Carmichael M, Brendler CB. Pathological and clinical findings to predict tumor extent of nonpalpable (stage T1c) prostate cancer. JAMA 1994;271:368–374.

54. Epstein JI, Steinberg GD. The significance of low-grade prostate cancer on needle biopsy. Cancer 1990;66:1927–1932.

55. Cupp MR, Bostwick DG, Myers RP, Oesterling JE. The volume of prostate cancer in the biopsy specimen cannot reliably predict the quantity of cancer in the radical prostatectomy specimen on an individual basis. J Urol 1995;153:1543–1548.

56. Irwin MB, Trapasso JG. Identification of insignificant prostate cancers: analysis of preoperative parameters. Urology 1994;44:862–868.

57. Peller PA, Young DC, Marmaduke DP, et al. Sextant prostate biopsies: a histopathologic correlation with radical prostatectomy specimens. Cancer 1995;75:530–538.

58. Bastacky SI, Walsh PC, Epstein JI. Relationship between perineural tumor invasion on needle biopsy and radical prostatectomy capsular penetration in clinical stage B adenocarcinoma of the prostate. Am J Surg Pathol 1993;17:336–341.

59. Villers A, McNeal JE, Redwine EA, et al. The role of perineural space invasion in local spread of prostatic adenocarcinoma. J Urol 1989;142:763–768.

60. Ostrowski ML, Wheeler TM. Paraganglia of the prostate: location, frequency, and differentiation from prostatic adenocarcinoma. Am J Surg Pathol 1994;18:412–420.

61. Brawer MK, Bigler SA, Sohlberg OE, et al. Significance of prostatic intraepithelial neoplasia on prostate needle biopsy. Urology 1991;38:103–107.

62. Weinstein MH, Epstein JI. Significance of high-grade prostatic intraepithelial neoplasia on needle biopsy. Hum Pathol 1993;24:624–629.

63. Ellis WJ, Brawer MK. Repeat prostate needle biopsy: who needs it? J Urol 1995;153:1496–1498.

64. Cantrell BB, DeKlerk DP, Eggleston JC, et al. Pathologic factors that influence prognosis in stage A prostatic cancer: the influence of extent versus grade. J Urol 1981;125:516–520.

65. Zhang G, Wasserman NF, Sidi AA, et al. Long-term followup results after expectant management of stage A1 prostatic cancer. J Urol 1991;146:99–103.

66. Epstein JI, Paull C, Eggelston JC, Walsh PC. Prognosis of untreated stage A1 prostatic carcinoma: a study of 94 cases with extended followup. J Urol 1986;136:837–839.

67. Blute ML, Zincke H, Farrow GM. Long-term followup of young patients with stage A adenocarcinoma of the prostate. J Urol 1986;136:840–843.

68. Larsen M, Ballentine Carter H, Epstein JI. Can stage A1 tumor extent be predicted by transurethral resection tumor volume, percent, or grade? A study of 64 stage A1 radical prostatectomies with comparison to prostates removed for stages A2 and B disease. J Urol 1991;164:1059–1063.

69. Lowe BA, Listrom MB. Management of stage A prostate cancer with a high probability of progression. J Urol 1988;140:1345–1347.

70. Lowe BA, Listrom MB. Incidental carcinoma of the prostate: an analysis of the predictors of progression. J Urol 1988;140:1340–1344.

71. Epstein JI, Oesterling JE, Walsh PC. Tumor volume versus percentage of specimen involved by tumor correlated with progression in stage A prostatic carcinoma. J Urol 1988;139:980–984.

72. Fan K, Peng CF. Predicting the probability of bone metastasis through histological grading of prostate carcinoma: a retrospective correlative analysis of 81 autopsy cases with antemortem transurethral resection specimens. J Urol 1983;130:708–711.

73. Humphrey P, Vollmer RT. The ratio of prostate chips with cancer. Hum Pathol 1988;19:411–418.

74. Mostofi FK. Prostate sampling. Am J Surg Pathol 1986;10:175. Editorial.

75. Humphrey PA, Walther PJ. Adenocarcinoma of the prostate: I. tissue sampling considerations. Am J Clin Pathol 1993;99:746–759.

76. Murphy WM, Dean PJ, Brasfield JA, Tatum L. Incidental carcinoma of the prostate. Am J Surg Pathol 1986;10:170–174.

77. Rohr LR. Incidental adenocarcinoma in transurethral resections of the prostate. Am J Surg Pathol 1987;11:53–58.

78. Vollmer RT. Prostate cancer and chip specimens: complete vs. partial sampling. Hum Pathol 1986;17:285–290.

79. McDowell PR, Fox WM, Epstein JI. Is submission of remaining tissue necessary when incidental carcinoma of the prostate is found on transurethral resection? Hum Pathol 1994;25:493–497.

80. Moore GH, Lawshe B, Murphy J. Diagnosis of adenocarcinoma in transurethral resectates of the prostate gland. Am J Surg Pathol 1986;10:165–169.

81. McNeal JE. Morphogenesis of prostatic carcinoma. Cancer 1965;18:1659–1666.

82. Helpap B. The biologic significance of atypical hyperplasia of the prostate. Virchows Arch [A]. 1980;387:307–317.

83. Kastendieck H. Correlations between atypical primary hyperplasia and carcinoma of the prostate. Pathol Res Pract 1980;169:366–387.

84. Kovi J, Jackson MA, Heshmat MY. Ductal spread in prostatic carcinoma. Cancer 1985;56:1566–1573.

85. Oyashu R, Bahnson RR, Nowels K, Garnett JE. Cytological atypia in the prostate gland: frequency, distribution and possible relevance to carcinoma. J Urol 1986;135:959–962.

86. McNeal JE, Bostwick DG. Intraductal dysplasia: a premalignant lesion of the prostate. Hum Pathol 1986;17:64–71.

87. Drago JR, Mostofi FK, Lee F. Introductory remarks and workshop summary: workshop on prostatic intraepithelial neoplasia, significance and correlation with prostate specific antigen and transrectal ultrasound. Urology 1989;34:2.

88. Bostwick DG, Brawer MK. Prostatic intra-epithelial neoplasia and early invasion in prostate cancer. Cancer 1987;59:788–794.

89. Kovi J, Mostofi FK, Hesmat MY, Enterline JP. Large acinar atypical hyperplasia and carcinoma of the prostate. Cancer 1988;61:555–561.

90. Troncoso P, Babaian RJ, Ro JY, et al. Prostatic intraepithelial neoplasia and invasive prostatic adenocarcinoma in cystoprostatectomy specimens. Urology 1989;34:52.

91. Quinn BD, Cho KR, Epstein JI. Relationship of severe dysplasia to stage B adenocarcinoma of the prostate. Cancer 1990;65:2328–2337.

92. McNeal JE, Villers A, Redwine RA, et al. Microcarcinoma in the prostate: its association with duct-acinar dysplasia. Hum Pathol 1991;22:644–652.

93. Montironi R, Braccishi A, Matera G, et al. Quantitation of the prostatic intra-epithelial neoplasia. Pathol Res Pract 1991;187:307–314.

94. Petein M, Michel P, Van Velthoven R, et al. Morphonuclear relationship between prostatic intraepithelial neoplasia and cancers as assessed by digital cell image analysis. Am J Clin Pathol 1991;96:628–634.

95. Montironi R, Scarpelli M, Sisti S, et al. Quantitative analysis of prostatic intraepithelial neoplasia on tissue sections. Anal Quant Cytol Histol 1990;12:366–372.

96. Berner A, Danielsen HE, Pettersen EO, et al. DNA distribution in the prostate. Anal Quant Cytol Histol 1993;15:247–252.

97. Amin MB, Schultz DS, Zarbo RJ, et al. Computerized static DNA ploidy analysis of prostatic intraepithelial neoplasia. Arch Pathol Lab Med 1993;117:794–798.

98. Crissman JD, Sakr WA, Hussein ME, Pontes JE. DNA quantitation of intraepithelial neoplasia and invasive carcinoma of the prostate. Prostate 1993;22:155–162.

99. Sakr WA, Haas GP, Cassin BF, et al. The frequency of carcinoma and intraepithelial neoplasia of the prostate in young male patients. J Urol 1993;150:379–385.

100. Melicow MM, Pachter MR. Endometrial carcinoma of prostatic utricle (uterus masculinus). Cancer 1967;20:1715–1722.

101. Melicow MM, Tannenbaum M. Endometrial carcinoma of the uterus masculinus (prostatic utricle): report of 6 cases. J Urol 1971;106:892–902.

102. Dube VE, Farrow GM, Greene LF. Prostatic adenocarcinoma of ductal origin. Cancer 1973;32:402–409.

103. Bostwick DG, Kindrachuk RW, Rouse RV. Prostatic adenocarcinoma with endometrioid features. Am J Surg Pathol 1985;9:595–609.

104. Epstein JI, Woodruff JM. Adenocarcinoma of the prostate with endometrioid features. Cancer 1986;57:111–119.

105. McNeal JE, Alroy J, Villers A, et al. Mucinous differentiation in prostatic adenocarcinoma. Hum Pathol 1991;22:979–988.

106. Epstein JI, Lieberman PH. Mucinous adenocarcinoma of the prostate gland. Am J Surg Pathol 1985;9:299–308.

107. Ro JY, Grignon DJ, Ayala AG, et al. Mucinous adenocarcinoma of the prostate. Hum Pathol 1990;21:593–600.

108. Remmele W, Weber A, Harding P. Primary signet-ring cell carcinoma of the prostate. Hum Pathol 1988;19:478–480.

109. Ro JY, El-Naggar A, Ayala AG, et al. Signet-ring cell carcinoma of the prostate. Am J Surg Pathol 1988;12:453–460.

110. Cohen R, Glezerson G, Taylor L, et al. The neuroendocrine cell population of the human prostate gland. J Urol 1993;150:365–368.

111. Di Sant'Agnese PA, De Mesy Jensen, KL. Neuroendocrine differentiation in prostatic carcinoma. Hum Pathol 1987;18:849–856.

112. Abrahamsson PA, Wadstrom LB, Alumets J, et al. Peptide-, hormone- and sertonin-immunoreactive tumour cells in carcinoma of the prostate. Pathol Res Pract 1987;182:298–307.

113. Abrahamsson PA, Falkmer S, Falt K, Grimelius L. The course of neuroendocrine differentiation in prostatic carcinomas. Pathol Res Pract 1989;185:373–380.

114. Di Sant'Agnese PA. Neuroendocrine differentiation in human prostatic carcinoma. Hum Pathol 1992;23:287–296.

115. Di Sant'Agnese PA. Neuroendocrine differentiation in carcinoma of the prostate. Cancer 1992;70:254–268.

116. Di Sant'Agnese PA. Neuroendocrine differentiation in prostatic carcinoma. Cancer 1995;75:1850–1859.

117. Aprikian AG, Cordon-Cardo C, Fair WR, Reuter VE. Characterization of neuroendocrine differentiation in human benign prostate and prostatic adenocarcinoma. Cancer 1993;71:3952–3965.

118. Aprikian AG, Cordon-Cardo C, Fair WR, et al. Neuroendocrine differentiation in metastatic prostatic adenocarcinoma. J Urol 1994;151: 914–919.

119. Cohen RJ, Glezerson G, Haffejee Z. Neuro-endocrine cells: a new prognostic parameter in prostate cancer. Br J Urol 1991;68:258–262.

120. Schron DS, Gipson T, Mendelsohn G. The histogenesis of small cell carcinoma of the prostate: an immunohistochemical study. Cancer 1984;53:2478–2480.

121. Oesterling JE, Hauzeur CG, Farrow GM. Small cell anaplastic carcinoma of the prostate: a clinical, pathological and immunohistological study of 27 patients. J Urol 1992;147:804–807.

122. Feiner HD, Gonzalez R. Carcinoma of the prostate with atypical immunohistochemical features. Am J Surg Pathol 1986;10:765–770.

123. Ro JY, Tetu B, Ayala AG, Ordonez NG. Small cell carcinoma of the prostate. Cancer 1987;59:977–982.

124. Tetu B, Ro JY, Ayala AG, et al. Small cell carcinoma of the prostate, part I. Cancer 1987;59:1803–1809.

125. Hindson DA, Knight LJ, Ocker JM. Small-cell carcinoma of the prostate. Urology 1985;26:182–184.

126. Amato RJ, Logothetis CJ, Hallinan R, et al. Chemotherapy for small cell carcinoma of prostatic origin. J Urol 1992;147:935–937.

127. Cleary KR, Choi HY, Ayala AG. Basal cell hyperplasia of the prostate. Am J Clin Pathol 1983;80:850–854.

128. Epstein JI, Armas OA. Atypical basal cell hyperplasia of the prostate. Am J Surg Pathol 1992;16:1205–1214.

129. Devaraj LT, Bostwick DG. Atypical basal cell hyperplasia of the prostate. Am J Surg Pathol 1993;17:645–659.

130. Frankel K, Craig JR. Adenoid cystic carcinoma of the prostate. Am J Clin Pathol 1974;62:639–645.

131. Tannenbaum M. Adenoid cystic or "salivary gland" carcinomas of the prostate. Urology 1975;6:238–239.

132. Lin JI, Garcia MB, Cohen EL, et al. Basal cell adenoma of the prostate. Urology 1978;11:409–410.

133. Kramer SA, Bredael JJ, Krueger RP. Adenoid cystic carcinoma of the prostate: report of a case. J Urol 1978;120:383–384.

134. Shong-san C, Walters MNI. Adenoid cystic carcinoma of prostate. Pathology 1984;16:337–338.

135. Kuhajda FP, Mann RB. Adenoid cystic carcinoma of the prostate. Am J Clin Pathol 1984;81:257–260.

136. Young RH, Frierson HF, Mills SE, et al. Adenoid cystic-like tumor of the prostate gland. Am J Clin Pathol 1988;89:49–56.

137. Denholm JW, Webb JN, Howard GCW, Chisholm GD. Basaloid carcinoma of the prostate gland: histogenesis and review of the literature. Histopathology 1992;20:151–155.

138. Cohen RJ, Goldberg RD, Verhaart MJS, Cohen M. Adenoid cyst-like carcinoma of the prostate gland. Arch Pathol Lab Med 1993;117: 799–801.

139. Reed RJ. Consultation case. Am J Surg Pathol 1984;8:699–704.

140. Shannon RL, Ro JY, Grignon DJ, et al. Sarcomatoid carcinoma of the prostate. Cancer 1992;69:2676–2682.

141. Wick MR, Young RH, Malvesta R, et al. Prostatic carcinosarcomas. Am J Clin Pathol 1989;92:131–139.

142. Forsslund G, Pier-Luigi E, Nilsson B, Zetterber A. The prognostic significance of nuclear DNA content in prostatic carcinoma. Cancer 1992;69:1432–1439.

143. Adolfsson J, Ronstrom L, Hedlund PO, et al. The prognostic value of modal deoxyribonucleic acid in low grade, low stage untreated prostate cancer. J Urol 1990;144:1404–1407.

144. Falkmer UG. Methodologic sources of errors in image and flow cytometric DNA assessments of the malignancy potential of prostatic carcinoma. Hum Pathol 1992;23:360–367.

145. Shankey TV, Kallioniemi OP, Koslowski JM, et al. Consensus review of the clinical utility of DNA content cytometry in prostate cancer. Cytometry 1993;14:497–500.

146. Epstein JI, Pizov G, Steinberg GD, et al. Correlation of prostate cancer nuclear deoxyribonucleic acid, size, shape, and Gleason grade with pathologic stage at radical prostatectomy. J Urol 1992;148:87–91.

147. Hardt NS, Hendricks JB, Sapi Z, et al. Ploidy results in prostatic carcinoma vary with sampling method and with cytometric technique. Mod Pathol 1994;7:44–48.

148. O'Malley FP, Grignon DJ, Keeney M, et al. DNA heterogeneity in prostatic adenocarcinoma. Cancer 1993;71:2797–2802.

149. Frankfurt OS, Chin JL, Englander LS, et al. Relationship between DNA ploidy, glandular differentiation, and tumor spread in human prostate cancer. Cancer Res 1985;45:1418–1423.

150. Dejter SW, Cunningham RE, Noguchi PD, et al. Prognostic signifi-

cance of DNA ploidy in carcinoma of the prostate. Urology 1989;33:361–366.

151. Baldalament RA, O'Toole RV, Young DC, Drago JR. DNA ploidy and prostate-specific antigen as prognostic factors in clinically resectable prostate cancer. Cancer 1991;67:3014–3023.

152. Greene DR, Taylor SR, Wheeler TM, Scardino PT. DNA ploidy by image analysis of individual foci of prostate cancer: a preliminary report. Cancer Res 1991;51:4084–4089.

153. Hussain MH, Powell I, Zaki N, et al. Flow cytometric DNA analysis of fresh prostatic resections. Cancer 1993;72:3012–3019.

154. Scrivner DL, Meyer JS, Rujanavech N, et al. Cell kinetics by bromode-oxyuridine labeling and deoxyribonucleic acid ploidy in prostatic carcinoma needle biopsies. J Urol 1991;146:1034–1039.

155. Tavares AS, Costa J, de Carvalho A, Reis M. Tumour ploidy and prognosis in carcinomas of the bladder and prostate. Br J Cancer 1966;20:438–441.

156. Peters-Gee JM, Miles BJ, Cerny JC, et al. Prognostic significance of DNA quantitation in stage D1 prostate carcinoma with the use of image analysis. Cancer 1992;70:1159–1165.

157. Tinari N, Natoli C, Angelucci D, et al. DNA and s-phase fraction analysis by flow cytometry in prostate cancer. Cancer 1993;1289–1296.

158. Van den Ouden D, Tribukait B, Blom JHM, et al. Deoxyribonucleic acid ploidy of core biopsies and metastatic lymph nodes of prostate cancer patients: impact on time to progression. J Urol 1993;150:400–406.

159. Song J, Cheng WS, Cupps RE, et al. Nuclear deoxyribonucleic acid content measured by static cytometry: important prognostic association for patients with clinically localized prostate carcinoma treated by external beam radiotherapy. J Urol 1992;147:794–797.

160. McIntire TL, Murphy WM, Coon JS, et al. The prognostic value of DNA ploidy combined with histologic substaging for incidental carcinoma of the prostate gland. Am J Clin Pathol 1988;89:370.

161. Peters JM, Miles BJ, Kubus JJ, Crissman JD. Prognostic significance of the nuclear DNA content in localized prostatic adenocarcinoma. Anal Quant Cytol Histol 1990;12:359–365.

162. Lundberg A, Carstensen J, Rundquist I. DNA flow cytometry and histopathological grading of paraffin-embedded prostate biopsy specimens in a survival study. Cancer Res 1987;47:1973–1977.

163. Fordham MVP, Burdge AH, Matthews J, et al. Prostatic carcinoma cell DNA content measured by flow cytometry and its relation to clinical outcome. Br J Surg 1986;73:400–403.

164. Lee SE, Currin SM, Paulson DF, Walther PJ. Flow cytometric determination of ploidy in prostatic adenocarcinoma: a comparison with seminal vesicle involvement and histopathological grading as a predictor of clinical recurrence. J Urol 1988;140:769–774.

165. Lieber MM, Murtaugh PA, Farrow GM, et al. DNA ploidy and surgically treated prostate cancer. Cancer 1995;75:1935–1943.

166. Carmichael MJ, Veltri RW, Partin AW, et al. Deoxyribonucleic acid ploidy analysis as a predictor of recurrence following radical prostatectomy for stage T2 disease. J Urol 1995;153:1015–1019.

167. Ritchie AWS, Dorey F, Layfield LJ, et al. Relationship of DNA content to conventional prognostic factors in clinically localized carcinoma of the prostate. Br J Urol 1988;62:254–260.

168. Humphrey PA, Walther PJ, Currin SM, Vollmer RT. Histologic grade, DNA ploidy, and intraglandular tumor extent as indicators of tumor progression of clinical stage B prostatic carcinoma. Am J Surg Pathol 1991;15:1165–1170.

169. Isaacs WB, Bova S, Morton RA, et al. Molecular genetics and chromosomal alterations in prostate cancer. Cancer 1995;75:2004–2012.

170. Sandberg AA. Chromosomal abnormalities and related events in prostate cancer. Hum Pathol 1992;23:368–380.

171. Stearns ME, McGarvey T. Prostate cancer: therapeutic, diagnostic, and basic studies. Lab Invest 1992;67:540–551.

172. Bookstein R. Tumor suppressor genes in prostatic oncogenesis. J Cell Biochem 1994;19(suppl):217–223.

173. Dong J-T, Lamb PW, Rinker-Schaeffer CW, et al. KAI1, a metastasis suppressor gene for prostate cancer on human chromosome 11p11.2. Science 1995;268:884–886.

174. Hinds PW, Weinberg RA. Tumor suppressor genes. Curr Opin Genet Dev 1994;4:135–141.

175. Thomas DJ, Robinson M, King P, et al. p53 expression and clinical outcome in prostate cancer. Br J Urol 1993;72:778–781.

176. Navone NM, Troncoso P, Pisters LL, et al. p53 protein accumulation and gene mutation in the progression of human prostate carcinoma. J Natl Cancer Inst 1993;85:1657–1667.

177. Watanabe M, Ushijima T, Kakiuchi H, et al. p53 gene mutations in human prostate cancers in Japan: different mutation spectra between Japan and Western countries. Jpn J Cancer Res 1994;85:904–910.

178. Effert PJ, McCoy RH, Walther PJ, Liu ET. p53 gene alteration in human prostate carcinoma. J Urol 1993;150:257–261.

179. Ittmann M, Wieczorek R, Heller P, et al. Alterations in the p53 and MDM-2 genes are infrequent in clinically localized, stage B prostate adenocarcinomas. Am J Pathol 1994;145:287–293.

180. Dinjens WN, van der Weiden MM, Schroeder FH, et al. Frequency and characterization of p53 mutations in primary and metastatic human prostate cancer. Int J Cancer 1994;56:630–633.

181. Myers RB, Oelschlager D, Srivastava S, Grizzle WE. Accumulation of the p53 protein occurs more frequently in metastatic than in localized prostatic adenocarcinomas. Prostate 1994;25:243–248.

182. Hall MC, Navone NM, Troncoso P, et al. Frequency and characterization of p53 mutations in clinically localized prostate cancer. Urology 1995;45:470–475.

183. Aprikian AG, Sarkis AS, Fair WR, et al. Immunohistochemical determination of p53 protein nuclear accumulation in prostatic adenocarcinoma. J Urol 1994;151:1276–1280.

184. Shurbaji MS, Kalbfleisch JH, Thurmond TS. Immunohistochemical detection of p53 protein as a prognostic indicator in prostate cancer. Hum Pathol 1995;106–109.

185. Sadasivan R, Morgan R, Jennings S, et al. Overexpression of HER-2/neu may be an indicator of poor prognosis in prostate cancer. J Urol 1993;150:126–131.

186. Kuhn EJ, Kurnot RA, Sesterhenn IA, et al. Expression of the c-erbB-2 (HER-2/neu) oncoprotein in human prostatic carcinoma. J Urol 1993;150:1427–1433.

187. Bushman EC, Nayak RN, Bushman W. Immunohistochemical staining of ras p21: staining in benign and malignant prostate tissue. J Urol 1995;153:233–237.

188. Taplin ME, Bubley GJ, Shuster TD, et al. Mutation of the androgen-receptor gene in metastatic androgen-independent prostate cancer. New Engl J Med 1995;332:1393–1398.

The Staging of ProstateCancer

▼   ▼   ▼   ▼   ▼   ▼   ▼   ▼

3

Anthony V. D'Amico
Francis T. McGovern
Paul A. Church
Clare M. C. Tempany

THE initial clinical staging system for adenocarcinoma of the prostate was proposed by Whitmore and Jewett in 1975 (1) (Table 3.1) and completely depended on the clinical findings on digital rectal examination (DRE) or the pathologic findings at a transurethral resection of the prostate (TURP). Gleason scoring, however,

Table 3.1 *Whitmore-Jewett clinical staging system for adenocarcinoma of the prostate*

Clinical Stage	Clinical Findings
A1[a]	Limited extent occult
A2[a]	Diffuse occult or poor differentiation
B1[b]	Induration < one lobe
B2[b]	Induration > one lobe
C1[b]	Minimal tumor; extraprostatic extension
C2[b]	Bulky tumor; extraprostatic extension
D0[b]	Tumor localized to the gland; elevated acid phosphatase
D1	Involved pelvic lymph nodes; no other metastasis
D2	Distant metastasis

[a]Clinical findings are from transurethral resection of the prostate.
[b]Clinical findings are from digital rectal examination.

▼

Table 3.2 *American Joint Commission on Cancer staging system for adenocarcinoma of the prostate*

Primary Tumor (T)

TX Primary tumor cannot be assessed

T0 No evidence of the primary tumor

T1 Clinically inapparent tumor not palpable nor visible by imaging

    T1a Tumor is an incidental histologic finding in ≤5% of tissue resected

    T1b Tumor is an incidental histologic finding in >5% of tissue resected

    T1c Tumor identified by needle biopsy on the basis of an elevated PSA

T2 Tumor confined to the prostate

    T2a Tumor involves ≤0.5 of a lobe

    T2b Tumor involves >0.5 of a lobe but not both lobes

    T2c Tumor involves both lobes

T3 Tumor extends through the prostatic capsule

    T3a Unilateral extracapsular extension

    T3b Bilateral extracapsular extension

    T3c Seminal vesicle involvement

T4 Tumor is fixed or invades adjacent structures other than the seminal vesicles

    T4a Tumor invades bladder neck, external sphincter, or rectum

    T4b Tumor invades levator muscles and/or is fixed to the pelvic sidewall

Regional Lymph Nodes (N)

NX Regional nodes cannot be assessed

N0 No regional lymph node metastasis

N1 Metastasis in a single lymph node, ≤2 cm in greatest dimension

N2 Metastasis in a single lymph node, >2 cm and ≤5 cm in greatest dimension, or in multiple lymph nodes, none >5 cm

N3 Metastasis in a lymph node, >5 cm in greatest dimension

Distant Metastasis (M)

MX Presence of distant metastasis cannot be assessed

M0 No distant metastasis

M1 Distant metastasis

    M1a Nonregional lymph node(s)

    M1b Bone(s)

    M1c Other site(s)

which on multivariate analysis has been shown to be superior in the prediction of long-term survival compared with clinical stage, was first incorpo-rated into the staging system by the American Joint Committee on Cancer (AJCC) in 1988 (2) and is included in the most recent staging system published by the AJCC in 1992 (Table 3.2).

Prostate-specific antigen (PSA) is now approved by the National Cancer Institute to be used in conjunction with the DRE for routine screening of prostate cancer in men 50 years old or older and has been shown to be the *most important* clinical indicator on multivariate analysis in predicting overall survival after definitive treatment for *clinical organ-confined prostate cancer* (3). Yet the PSA is not included in the current staging systems.

Other experimental modalities that may lead to improved clinical staging of clinical organ-confined prostate cancer include the endorectal coil magnetic resonance imaging study (4), and a molecular biology technique that allows for the detection of circulating prostate cancer cells in the peripheral blood, called the polymerase chain reaction (PCR) (5). In this section, an examination of all the relevant clinical parameters that can be used in the clinical staging of prostate cancer is offered, to provide a framework in which to classify prostate cancer patients that will serve as the basis for optimizing management decisions.

■ **THE DIGITAL RECTAL EXAMINATION**

What Is the Prognostic Significance of the Clinical Findings on the Digital Rectal Examination?

Since the advent of PSA-based screening, more patients are presenting with smaller volume tumors and nonpalpable (stage T1c) disease (6). In the past and up until the late 1980s, clinical stage was an important prognostic indicator after treatment with either surgery or radiation therapy. Today the digital rectal exam is still a strong negative prognostic indicator in the setting of a clinical stage T3 tumor with marked extraprostatic disease—either in the form of seminal vesicle invasion (SVI) or gross transcapsular extension (TCE) of disease—or in the case of a clinical stage T4 prostate with disease fixed to juxtaposed structures (i.e., rectum, bladder) (7). However, for patients with clinical organ-confined or nonpalpable disease, clinical stage is the least important predictor on multivariate analysis when testing for the outcomes of TCE or SVI at the time of radical prostatectomy or for identifying patients who will enjoy long-term PSA-failure-free survival after definitive local management (8).

What Is Combined Modality Staging?

Based on the observation that patients with pathologic organ-confined disease at the time of radical prostatectomy are the most likely to achieve long-term survival, followed by patients with microscopic extracapsular extension, established transcapsular extension, seminal vesicle involvement, and, finally, in the worse prognostic category, positive pelvic lymph nodes (9), a more accurate pre-therapy staging system could optimize the initial therapeutic approach. Combined modality staging is a methodology in which all of the pretreatment clinical factors that have independent prognostic significance on multivariate analysis for predicting pathologic organ-confined disease are used to determine the optimal initial management. The first investigators to publish such an algorithm were Partin and colleagues at Johns Hopkins University (8). They found independent prognostic significance for the prostate-specific antigen, biopsy Gleason sum, and clinical stage in predicting pathologic evidence of TCE and SVI for patients with clinical organ-confined disease (clinical stage T1 or T2). Moreover, they found that the strongest pathologic predictor of both TCE and SVI was the PSA, followed by the biopsy Gleason grade and finally the clinical stage as per the digital rectal examination. At the University of Pennsylvania, D'Amico and colleagues (10) performed a similar analysis using, in addition to the PSA, biopsy Gleason sum, and clinical stage, the endorectal coil magnetic resonance imaging results. Their findings are similar to Partin's in that, again, the PSA was the most important predictor of clinically occult extraprostatic disease. The endorectal coil MRI, however, was second, and the biopsy Gleason sum third in predicting for occult TCE or SVI, whereas the clinical stage was not a significant independent predictor.

When trying to predict the metastatic potential of a tumor, the grade (Gleason score) is the most significant prognostic factor, verified by the fact that Gleason score is the most significant predictor of pelvic lymph node involvement, as confirmed by Partin and colleagues (8) and others (11). The most commonly used system to describe the tumor grade is the Gleason score, which recognizes the heterogeneity of prostate cancer. The two most predominant histologic patterns are assigned a value from 1 (well differentiated) through 5 (poorly differentiated), and the sum of those two values represents the Gleason score. Local regional extent of disease, however (i.e., TCE, SVI), is best assessed by the pathologic tumor volume. Tumor volume has been correlated with both the serum PSA as shown by Stamey (12) (correlation coefficient of PSA and tumor volume = 0.7), and the number of positive biopsies on a routine sextant biopsy (13). Tumors with a volume less than 4 cc are usually organ confined, while those larger than 12 cc are essentially always associated with metastatic disease.

■ IS RADIOLOGIC STAGING REQUIRED PRIOR TO LOCAL THERAPY?

When the ultrasound-guided biopsy reveals carcinoma, the responsible physician caring for the newly diagnosed prostate cancer patient must make an assessment—based on the available information (DRE, PSA, Gleason score)—as to whether further radiologic staging is necessary. In asymptomatic patients who are in a favorable prognostic group (PSA ≤10 ng/mL, biopsy Gleason score ≤6, and clinical stage T1a,b,c or T2a), further radiologic staging is *not routinely recommended* prior to local therapy. In less favorable patients (PSA >10 ng/mL, biopsy Gleason score ≥7, or clinical stage T2b or higher), further radiologic staging *may be helpful*.

In particular, radiologic imaging modalities were disappointing until the advent of the endorectal coil MRI for predicting extent of local disease. In a large population-based screening study with 6,987 patients, performed by Keetch and collaborators (14), only one-third of the hypoechoic lesions seen on transrectal ultrasound (TRUS) were in fact positive on biopsy, whereas two-thirds of the normal-appearing glands on TRUS contained cancer as confirmed by biopsy. In a prospective randomized study performed by the Radiology Diagnostic Oncology Group, a comparison of *body coil* MRI and TRUS for determining clinically nonpalpable extraprostatic disease found no significant difference, with an approximate 60% accuracy overall (15). Single-institution series of CT pelvis scans have shown similar disappointing results, with about 60% accuracy in detecting extraprostatic disease in clinical stage A and B patients. Single-institution series on the accuracy of the *endorectal coil* MRI have claimed an encouraging 70% to 80% accuracy in predicting pathologic stage C tumors in clinical stage A and B patients (10,16,17). These studies are in agreement with the University of Pennsylvania data that predict 72% accuracy (70% for TCE, 88% for SVI) in the detection of clinically occult extraprostatic disease based solely on the endorectal coil MRI study (10). Endorectal coil MRI can image the prostate in three orthogonal planes (transverse, sagittal, coronal), and the glandular anatomy is well defined on T2-weighted images. Prostate cancer is typically a focal area of low signal intensity seen predominately in the periphery (outer two-thirds) of the prostate on T2-weighted MR images. These areas are not 100% specific for cancer, however, in that some types of benign prostatic hypertrophy and prostatitis can appear similar.

Categorization of PSA Failure After Definitive Local Therapy Using Combined Modality Staging

Table 3.3 shows the two-year actuarial freedom from PSA failure rates among 463 patients treated with a radical prostatectomy for clinically organ-confined prostate cancer at the University of Pennsylvania (18). As expected, for patients with a PSA greater than 4 to 10 ng/mL and well-differentiated tumors (biopsy Gleason sum 2 to 4) or patients with a PSA less than 4 and a biopsy Gleason sum less than or equal to 6, the two-year actuarial freedom from biochemical failure rate is high (98%). Moreover, the pathologic organ confinement rate is correspondingly high, being at least 84% in this select group of patients, which represents about 15% of all patients in today's screened population. Conversely, the poor prognosis patients who, despite clinical organ-confined disease, have two-year actuarial freedom from PSA failure rates of at most 32% are those patients with a pretreatment serum PSA greater than 20 ng/mL or poorly differentiated tumor (Gleason sum ≥8) found on biopsy. As

Table 3.3 *Pretreatment clinical characteristics, corresponding pathologic organ confinement rate, and two-year actuarial PSA failure rate for 463 prostate cancer patients treated with radical retropubic prostatectomy*

Clinical Pretreatment Characteristics	Pathologic Organ-Confined Disease (%)	Two-year Freedom from PSA Failure (%)
Low Risk		
PSA 0–4; Gleason* 2–6	84	98
PSA >4–10; Gleason 2–4	88	98
Intermediate Risk		
PSA >4–10; Gleason 5–7	70	80
PSA 0–4; Gleason 7		
PSA >10–20; Gleason 2–7	57	68
High Risk		
PSA >20	30	27
Gleason ≥8	28	32

*Gleason = biopsy Gleason sum.

expected, pathologic organ-confined disease is present in this group in at most 30% of the cases, and this population accounts for about 15% of all prostate cancer patients.

The remaining patients comprise the intermediate risk group, accounting for approximately ⅔ of all PSA-based patients. These patients were found to have pathologic organ-confined disease in 57% to 70% of cases, with a resulting 68% to 80% two-year actuarial freedom from PSA failure. In this patient group, the endorectal coil MRI data were able to stratify patients into high and low risk for postoperative PSA failure by identifying clinically occult seminal vesicle invasion or transcapsular disease. Specifically, for patients with the following

1. PSA greater than 4 to 10 ng/mL and biopsy Gleason sum 5 to 7.
2. PSA 0 to 4 ng/mL and biopsy Gleason sum 7.
3. PSA greater than 10 to 20 ng/mL and biopsy Gleason sum 2 to 7.

a positive endorectal coil MRI for either SVI or TCE was predictive of a three-year actuarial freedom from postoperative PSA failure rate of at most 35%. Those patients with a negative endorectal coil MRI had three-year actuarial freedom from PSA failure rates of at least 80% as shown in Figures 3.1 and 3.2. Although these data are from a single institution and await verification from other investigators, the endorectal coil MRI may become the premiere staging study for this subgroup. At the current time, however, the study is not routinely recommended.

In summary, the serum PSA, biopsy Gleason sum, and, in some select cases, the endorectal coil MRI may provide a combined modal-

```
        PSA    0-4,  b Gleason 7
        PSA > 4-10,  b Gleason 5-7
        PSA >10-20,  b Gleason 2-7


%      100  +X......O.
         -       X.O.OOOO.O..
s̄        -          X..X...  O.OO.OOO.
         -              X..         O.............
P        -             X...X..
S        -                 X.....
A        -                             .
       50  +                          X.
F        -                            X.
A        -                            X...........
I        -                                            .
L        -                                            X
U        -
R        -    p < .0001
E        0  +
           .+....+....+....+....+....+....+....+.
            0    5   10   15   20   25   30   35
```

TIME (months)

```
        X   MR + TCE
        O   MR - TCE
```

Fig. 3.1 *TCE: Freedom from PSA failure by actuarial calculation for patients with a preoperative PSA greater than 4–10 ng/mL and biopsy Gleason sum 5–7, preoperative PSA 0–4 ng/mL and biopsy Gleason sum 7, or preoperative PSA greater than 10–20 ng/mL and biopsy Gleason sum 2–7, stratified for the presence or absence of extracapsular extension of disease on endorectal coil MRI (p < 0.0001).*

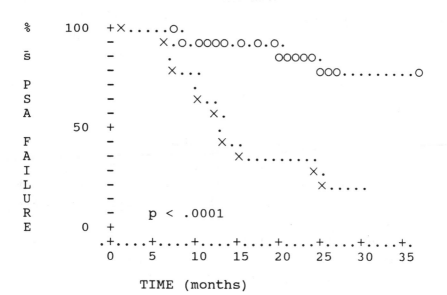

```
        PSA   0-4,  b Gleason 7
        PSA > 4-10, b Gleason 5-7
        PSA >10-20, b Gleason 2-7


 %    100  +X.....O.
      -           X.O.OOOO.O.O.O.
 s̄    -              .                OOOOO.
      -           X...                    OOO.........O
 P    -              .
 S    -            X..
 A    -             X.
      50  +            .
 F    -             X..
 A    -              X..........
 I    -                 X.
 L    -                 X.....
 U    -
 R    -      p < .0001
 E    0  +
        .+....+....+....+....+....+....+....+.
         0    5    10   15   20   25   30   35
```

                    TIME (months)

                X MR + SVI
                O MR - SVI
```

**Fig. 3.2** *SVI: Freedom from PSA failure by actuarial calculation for patients with a preoperative PSA greater than 4–10 ng/mL and biopsy Gleason sum 5–7, preoperative PSA 0–4 ng/mL and biopsy Gleason sum 7, or preoperative PSA greater than 10–20 ng/mL and biopsy Gleason sum 2–7, stratified for the presence or absence of seminal vesicle invasion on endorectal coil MRI (p < 0.0001).*

ity staging system far superior to any single variable alone for predicting occult extraprostatic disease in patients with clinical organ-confined disease as per the DRE.

### Can the Number of Positive Biopsies Obtained During a Sextant Sampling Predict for Extraprostatic Disease?

Investigators at the University of San Francisco (13) have conducted a multivariate analysis examining the number of positive biopsies from a standard sextant biopsy in conjunction with the serum PSA,
```

biopsy Gleason sum, and endorectal coil MRI findings to determine the presence of clinically occult TCE in patients with clinical organ-confined disease on the DRE. The small number of patients studied ($n = 57$) does not allow a definitive conclusion regarding the relative importance of the number of positive biopsies and endorectal coil MRI findings in predicting TCE; however, a trend ($p = 0.12$) in favor of MRI was noted. Larger studies are now ongoing to evaluate the impact that the number of positive biopsies will have on predicting for pathologic organ-confined disease.

■ DEFINING THE ROLE OF THE BONE SCAN

The purpose of the radionuclide bone scan is to assess the presence and extent of bony metastatic disease. Several large series (19,20) have shown a rare (<2%) positive bone scan in patients with clinical organ-confined disease, PSA less than 20 ng/mL, and a biopsy Gleason sum of 6 or less. As a result, the bone scan is no longer routinely required as a baseline study in this low-risk population of patients, in the absence of symptoms (bone pain) and a normal alkaline phosphatase.

Two large clinical studies have been conducted by investigators at the Mayo Clinic in an effort to use the serum PSA to eliminate the need for a staging radionuclide bone scan. The first study, conducted by Chybowski and colleagues (19), retrospectively analyzed 521 patients who presented to the Mayo Clinic between January 1987 and January 1989 with biopsy-proven prostate cancer. The results showed that all patients with PSA 10 ng/mL or less had a negative bone scan, with only 1% (1 of 99) of all patients with a PSA greater than 10 to 20 ng/mL having a positive bone scan. This was followed by a second investigation, conducted by Oesterling and colleagues (20), in which 852 patients with newly diagnosed adenocarcinoma of the prostate and PSA under 20 ng/mL were evaluated to ascertain the bone scan results. They found all patients with a PSA less than 8 ng/mL to have a negative bone scan. Only 3 patients (0.5%) with a PSA less than 10 ng/mL had a positive bone scan.

On the basis of the results of these two studies (19,20), Dr. Oesterling at the Mayo Clinic has recommended that a staging radionuclide bone scan is not necessary for patients who have newly diagnosed prostate cancer and no skeletal symptoms and whose PSA is less than 10 ng/mL.

■ THE ROLE OF PELVIC LYMPHADENECTOMY

Pelvic lymph node dissection provides the most accurate measure of assessing the pelvic lymph nodes (21). With the increased adaptation of laparoscopic lymph node dissection, or "minilaparotomy" open pelvic lymphadenectomy, morbidity has been reduced. Currently, the standard of care for lymph node–positive patients with a negative bone scan is to administer androgen ablative therapy. Therefore, lymph node dissection is primarily used to exclude patients from local therapy in the absence of local symptoms.

Because PSA has shifted the spectrum of prostate cancer to earlier disease presentation, only 7% of currently diagnosed patients who are surgical candidates are found to have involved pelvic lymph nodes (22). Several investigators have attempted to classify patients into high- and low-risk groups for involved pelvic lymph nodes on the basis of the clinical stage, PSA, and biopsy Gleason sum, thereby obviating the need for the lymph node sampling and its attendant morbidity. In particular, three independent surgical series (8,22,23) revealed that when clinical stage, PSA, and biopsy Gleason sum were used, a less than 5% risk of positive pelvic lymph nodes was noted in patients with clinical stage T1a, T1c, or T2a disease with a PSA under 20 ng/mL *and* a biopsy Gleason sum of 6 or less.

Therefore, for patients with PSA greater than 20 ng/mL or poorly differentiated tumors (biopsy Gleason sum ≥7), particularly those with clinical stage T2b tumor or higher who are to be managed with primary radiation therapy, a pelvic lymph node sampling should be considered to define the node-positive patients.

■ THE FUTURE

A molecular technique that allows for the detection in serum of a small amount of the messenger RNA that codes for PSA, called the polymerase chain reaction, has been developed. One study by Katz and colleagues (5) at Columbia University suggests that the PCR technique is capable of predicting clinically occult metastatic disease.

In this study, 39% of patients with clinically localized disease had positive PCR assays for PSA preoperatively. Of those patients with a positive PCR assay, 68% had TCE, 83% had SVI, and 87% had PSM at the time of pathologic sectioning of the radical prostatectomy specimen. Seiden and colleagues (24) at Harvard Medical School, using the same assay, found a direct correlation with a positive PCR test for PSA and the course of the disease. Specifically, 6%, 13%, and 50% of patients with clinically localized disease, hormone-responsive metastatic disease, and hormone-refractory metastatic disease had a positive PCR assay for PSA. Ghossein and colleagues (25) at Memorial Sloan-Kettering Cancer Center have reported that the PCR assay was positive in 6 of 16 patients (38%) with known metastatic prostate cancer on hormonal therapy. This study suggests that the PCR assay may be able to detect residual disease in patients on androgen ablative therapy thought to be in remission by biochemical criteria. All these studies with the PCR technique are preliminary but suggest that PCR may aid in identifying those patients with clinically occult but disseminated disease at presentation, in whom the use of both a local and a systemic therapy as initial management may impart a survival benefit. However, at this time both PCR and combining local and systemic therapy as the initial management for clinical organ-confined prostate cancer remain experimental. A test of this assay's ability to predict for clinically occult extraprostatic disease using a multivariate analysis in which all known prognostic factors are included will determine its role in the staging of clinical organ-confined prostate cancer patients.

Tumor microvessel density has recently been shown to correlate with a significantly worse four-year actuarial freedom from PSA and clinical failure after external beam radiation therapy (26). The study suggests that tumor angiogenesis may be prognostic for outcome after local therapy for clinical organ-confined prostate cancer because of its association with micrometastatic disease or a more advanced stage. Finally, other investigators (27) are examining whether the magnitude of the androgen receptor expression on the surface of prostate cancer cells predicts for long-term cure after local therapy.

■ CONCLUSION

The current staging system for adenocarcinoma of the prostate includes biopsy Gleason sum and digital rectal examination or transurethral resection findings. Obviously more recent parameters, including PSA, endorectal coil MRI, and the number of positive biopsies on a standard sextant biopsy, may add valuable information that can be used in guiding management decisions. Investigational tools such as PCR, tumor vascularity measurements, and androgen receptor quantification may lead to a further enhancement of our current ability to accurately define the pathologic extent of disease, but these tools await future testing on multivariate analysis against the established prognostic factors.

Combined modality staging as described in this chapter is a methodology that allows the physician to use all of the available and independently predictive information on multivariate analysis to guide the optimal initial therapy for patients with clinical organ-confined prostate cancer.

Editorial Comment

The reader should recognize that the staging of prostate cancer is not a uniform process throughout the country. What is considered adequate staging in one hospital or by one group of physicians may not be considered adequate by others.

The fundamental question that every physician treating a patient with prostate cancer wants answered is whether the cancer is confined to the prostate. As the authors mention, the Gleason score of the primary tumor is extremely important in predicting the extent of disease, and the Gleason score and serum PSA together are superior to either parameter considered alone.

To date, radiographic staging of the extent of local disease has been disappointing. Transrectal ultrasound, abdominal and pelvic CT scan, and body coil MRI have not been very helpful in predicting local tumor extension. The authors report a preliminary experience with endorectal coil MRI that is encouraging. However, the reader should recognize that not every hospital or physician has access to the endorectal coil, and that at present, Gleason score and serum PSA are the best and most widely used predictors of the extent of local disease.

The valuable study by Oesterling and colleagues from the Mayo Clinic argues persuasively that men with a serum PSA of 8 ng/mL or less are unlikely to have bone metastases, and that a bone scan may not be necessary in this group of patients.

■ **REFERENCES**

1. Jewett HJ. The present status of radical prostatectomy for stages A and B prostatic cancer. Urol Clin North Am 1975;2:105–124.
2. Beahrs OH, Henson DE, Hutter RVP, Kennedy BJ. American Joint Committee on Cancer: Manual for staging cancer. 4th ed. Philadelphia: JP Lippincott, 1992;181–186.
3. Zagars GK, Pollack A, Kavadi VS, Von Eschenbach A. Prostate-specific antigen and radiation therapy for clinically localized prostate cancer. Int J Radiat Oncol Biol Phys 1995;32:293–306.
4. Schnall MD, Bezzi M, Pollack HN, Kressel HY. Magnetic resonance imaging in the prostate. Magn Reson Imaging 1990;61:1–16.
5. Katz AE, Olsson CA, Raffo AJ, et al. Molecular staging of prostate cancer with the use of an enhanced reverse transcriptase-PCR assay. Urology 1994;43:765–775.
6. Catalona WJ, Smith DS, Ratliff TL, Basler JW. Detection of organ-confined prostate cancer is increased through prostate-specific-antigen–based screening. JAMA 1993;270:948–954.
7. Hanks GE. Optimizing the radiation treatment and outcome of prostate cancer. Int J Radiat Oncol Biol Phys 1985;11:1235–1245.
8. Partin AW, Yoo J, Ballentine Carter H, et al. The use of prostate specific antigen, clinical stage, and Gleason score to predict pathologic stage in men with prostate cancer. J Urol 1993;150:110–114.
9. Trapasso JG, DeKernion JB, Smith RB, Dorey F. The incidence and significance of detectable levels of serum prostate specific antigen after radical prostatectomy. J Urol 1994;152:1821–1825.
10. D'Amico AV, Whittington R, Malkowicz SB, et al. A multivariable analysis of clinical factors predicting for pathological features associated with local failure after radical prostatectomy for prostate cancer. Int J Radiat Oncol Biol Phys 1994;30:293–302.
11. Zagars GK, Ayala AG, von Eschenback AC, Pollack A. The prognostic significance of Gleason grade in prostatic adenocarcinoma: a long-term

follow-up study of 648 patients treated with radiation therapy. Int J Radiat Oncol Biol Phys 1995;31:237–245.

12. Stamey TA, Yang N, Hay AR, et al. Prostate-specific antigen as a serum marker for adenocarcinoma of the prostate. N Engl J Med 1987;317:909–916.

13. Presti JC, Katsuto S, Hricak H, et al. Clinical parameters in the preoperative evaluation for extracapsular extension at radical prostatectomy. American Urological Association Abstract 801, 1995:429A.

14. Keetch DW, Catalona WJ, Smith DS. Serial prostatic biopsies in men with persistently elevated serum prostate specific antigen values. J Urol 1994;151:1571–1574.

15. Rifkin MD, Zerhouni EA, Gatsonis CA, et al. Comparison of magnetic resonance imaging and ultrasonography in staging early prostate cancer: results of a multi-institutional cooperative trial. N Engl J Med 1990;323:621–626.

16. Chelsky MJ, Schnall MD, Seidmon JE, Pollack HM. Use of the endorectal surface coil magnetic resonance imaging for local staging of prostate cancer. J Urol 1993;150:391–395.

17. Krebs TL, Silverman JM. Clinical utility of endorectal surface coil imaging of the prostate gland. Radiol Soc North Am 1992;1006:275. Abstract.

18. D'Amico AV, Whittington R, Malkowicz SB, et al. A multivariate analysis of clinical and pathological factors which predict for prostate-specific antigen failure after radical prostatectomy after prostate cancer. J Urol 1995;154:131–138.

19. Chybowski FM, Larson-Keller JJ, Bergstralh EJ, et al. Predicting radionuclide bone scan findings in patients with newly diagnosed, untreated prostate cancer: prostate specific antigen is superior to all other clinical parameters. J Urol 1991;145:313–317.

20. Oesterling JE, Martin SK, Bergstralh EJ, et al. The use of prostate specific antigen in staging patients with newly diagnosed prostate cancer. JAMA 1993;269:57–64.

21. Danella JF, deKernion JB, Smith RB, Steckel J. The contemporary incidence of lymph node metastases in prostate cancer: implications for laparoscopic lymph node dissection. J Urol 1993;149:1488–1491.

22. Narayan P, Fournier G, Gajendran V, et al. Utility of preoperative prostate-specific antigen concentration and biopsy Gleason score in predicting risk of pelvic lymph node metastases in prostate cancer. Urology 1994;44:519–524.

23. Bishoff JT, Reyes A, Thompson IM, et al. Pelvic lymphadenectomy can

be omitted in selected patients with carcinoma of the prostate: development of a system of patient selection. Urology 1995;45:270–274.

24. Seiden MV, Kantoff PW, Krithivas K, et al. Detection of circulating tumor cells in men with localized or metastatic prostate cancer. J Clin Oncol 1994;12:2634–2639.

25. Ghossein RA, Scher HI, Gerald WL, et al. Detection of circulating tumor cells in patients with localized and metastatic prostatic carcinoma: clinical implications. J Clin Oncol 1995;13:1195–1200.

26. Hall MC, Troncoso P, Pollack A, et al. Significance of tumor angiogenesis in clinically localized prostate carcinoma treated with external beam radiotherapy. Urology 1994;44:869–875.

27. Ruizeveld de Winter JA, Janssen PJA, Sleddens HMEB, et al. Androgen receptor status in localized and locally progressive hormone refractory human prostate cancer. Am J Pathol 1994;144:735–746.

How to Use PSA in Managing Patients with Prostate Cancer

4

Anthony L. Zietman
Philip W. Kantoff
Kevin R. Loughlin

O NCE the diagnosis of prostate cancer has been made, a patient's prostate-specific antigen level remains a valuable tool. PSA level may be used to determine disease extent, to help select the most suitable therapy, and, once treatment has been completed, to flag a failure before it becomes clinically or symptomatically apparent.

■ PROSTATE SPECIFIC ANTIGEN (PSA): GENERAL CONSIDERATIONS

Prostate specific antigen (PSA) is a single chain glycoprotein that was first identified in the seminal plasma (1). It is produced by human prostatic epithelium (2) and its principal physiologic role appears to be liquefaction of the ejaculate (3). PSA is made by both benign and malignant prostate tissue (4), although approximately 10 times more PSA is made per gram of malignant tissue (5).

The role of PSA in prostate cancer screening is reviewed in another portion of the book, so we will not repeat it here. However certain concepts are worth brief review.

■ PSA VELOCITY

PSA velocity refers to the change of PSA levels over time, and as such is a misnomer; it would be more correctly termed PSA acceleration or

PSA slope. However PSA velocity has for some reason established a foothold in the prostate cancer literature (6). The concept of PSA velocity is based on the belief that PSA levels will rise more rapidly in patients with underlying prostate cancer than with benign disease. Carter et al (7) have reported that a PSA increase of greater than 0.75 ug/L per year is a useful indicator to help identify men with occult prostate cancer. However, the utility of PSA velocity is valid only if the PSA value is obtained at the same laboratory and by using the same PSA assay and methodology.

■ PSA DENSITY

The concept of PSA density is based again on the observation that both benign and malignant prostate tissue made PSA, but that malignant tissue makes more per gram. Therefore some men with benign prostate glands, particularly large prostates will have elevated PSA levels that do not signify prostate cancer. The measurement of prostate specific antigen density (PSAD) is derived by dividing the serum PSA level by the estimated prostate volume. The prostate volume is calculated by using the length, width and height of the prostate as measured by transrectal ultrasound and using the prolate ellipse formula, volume = $0.52 \times (L \times W \times H)$ (8).

The application of PSAD is most useful in patients with an intermediate elevation of serum PSA (4–10 ng/mL) who have a normal rectal exam. In this group, it has been recommended that patients with a PSAD (≥ 0.15) should undergo prostate needle biopsy (9). However not all investigators have found that PSAD enhances cancer detection (10). One concern is that the measurement of prostate volume may be somewhat user dependent. Another is that PSAD requires the patient to undergo an additional transrectal ultrasound exam which increases cost and patient discomfort.

■ AGE SPECIFIC PSA LEVELS

Age specific PSA levels have been developed in an attempt to make PSA levels more useful in detecting prostate cancer. The rationale behind PSA levels again lies in the fact that benign prostate tissue elaborates PSA. Therefore as men age and their prostate enlarges, one would expect their "background" PSA levels to increase. Using this hypotheses, Oesterling et al (11) studied a cohort of men in

Table 4.1 *Age Specific PSA Ranges*

Age (yrs.)	PSA value (ng/ml)
40–49	0–2.5
50–59	0–3.5
60–69	0–4.5
70–70	0–6.5

Minnesota and recommended the age specific values that appear in Table 1.

These ranges can be used to lower the PSA threshold to biopsy younger men while increasing the threshold to biopsy in older men.

■ **PSA ASSAYS**

There are now multiple commercially available serum assays used to determine PSA levels. Among the more commonly used are the Yang Pros Check, Abbott IMX, Tosoh AIA – PACK PA and Nichols Institute (12).

It is beyond the scope or intent of this chapter to critique or recommend the individual assays. What is important to communicate is that the assays have different methodologies and have different normal ranges. Therefore it is very important to know when comparing serial PSA levels in an individual patient, if the same assay was used and what the normal ranges are in the laboratory where the test was performed.

Once the diagnosis of prostate cancer has been made, PSA remains a valuable tool. Its level may be used to determine disease extent, help select the most suitable therapy, and, once treatment has been completed to flag a failure before it becomes clinically or symptomatically apparent.

■ **PSA AS A PROGNOSTIC INDICATOR**

For the newly diagnosed patient, the likelihood of having organ-confined disease is inversely proportional to the level of the PSA (13). As the PSA rises, the likelihood of having potentially curable prostate cancer decreases. Although there is no absolute level above which one can definitively say that incurable or metastatic prostate cancer exists, the likelihood of cure with some form of local therapy declines considerably once the PSA exceeds 15–20 ng/mL (14). At the time of diagnosis, however, the likelihood of showing visible metastatic disease on a bone scan is also proportional to the level of the PSA. The results of several studies have indicated that the likelihood of demonstrating a positive bone scan is rare for patients with PSA levels under 20 ng/mL and increases proportionately thereafter. The majority of patients with PSA levels greater than 100 ng/mL will simultaneously have positive bone scans.

A range of therapeutic possibilities are usually offered to the patient with the new diagnosis of prostate cancer. They are commonly laid out as if each were an equally valid option, and the patient may become confused if the decision is left to him. In truth, a review of the available pretreatment data can often be used to considerably narrow or refine the treatment options. PSA adds to clinical staging and biopsy Gleason grade in determining prognosis with therapy.

A number of surgical and radiation series have now been reported in which the results have been broken down by pretreatment PSA. It has become clear that cure by conventional external beam radiation is very rare once the PSA exceeds 20 ng/mL. Indeed the prognosis worsens considerably in most series once it exceeds 10 ng/mL (15–17). Those with serum PSA values in excees of 20 ng/mL commonly fail because of occult metastases not detected at the initial staging. However, those with PSA values between 10 and 20 ng/mL, if their Gleason sum is below 8, may well have too much disease at the primary site to sterilize with conventional external beam doses and techniques. These men might be better served either by surgery or by more advanced radiation techniques such as high-dose conformal therapy (18) or the modern radiation implant, perhaps in combination with external beam (19). Or they may be equally managed by prior cytoreduction with temporary "neo-adjuvant" androgen suppression before radiation (20). There is mounting evidence that this technique offers improved control rates at very little cost in additional morbidity. As such, it is probably better suited to smaller community hospitals than more risky high-dose radiation.

PSA can be used to predict the outcome of surgery and to guide patient counseling. When the serum PSA exceeds 20 ng/mL, the chance of cure with surgery alone is greatly reduced. Some series have suggested that as few as 50% will fail; others are more pessimistic, reporting more like 80%. These men should therefore be told that their chance for cure is low and may not justify the risks of surgery. Indeed many of the larger urologic centers concentrate their efforts on men with the highest chance of cure—that is, PSA less than 10 ng/mL and a Gleason sum of 7 or less. Alternatively, some form of combined modality therapy can be recommended, such as surgery with postoperative radiation if the margins are positive, or surgery with either neo-adjuvant or adjuvant androgen suppression.

PSA therefore may be used to guide the initial management of the patient. It determines who can be offered monotherapy with an optimistic chance of success, who with a lower chance for success, and who, if a curative approach is to be taken at all, will need combined modality therapy (Table 4.2).

Table 4.2 *How PSA may affect treatment options for a man with a medium-grade (Gleason 5–6) T1–2 adenocarcinoma of the prostate*

Pretreatment PSA (ng/mL)	Treatment Options
<10	Radical prostatectomy
	External beam radiation
	Radiation implant
10–20	Radical prostatectomy
	High-dose conformal external beam radiation
	Radiation implant + external beam
	Combined androgen suppression + radiation
20–30	Radical prostatectomy ± adjuvant radiation
	Combined androgen supression + radiation
>30	Combined androgen suppression + radiation
	Androgen suppression alone

SOURCE: Zietman AL, Shipley WU, Coen JJ. Radical prostatectomy and radical radiation therapy for clinical T_{1-2} adenocarcinoma of the prostate: new insights into outcome from rebiopsy and PSA follow-up. J Urol 1994;152:1806–1812.

■ THE EARLY DETECTION AND MANAGEMENT OF FAILURE

As the serum PSA is used routinely to detect de novo prostate cancer early, so it may also be used to detect failure of radical therapy at an early stage. This allows for

1. more rapid assessment of radical therapies than was previously possible with clinical end points alone.
2. the rapid institution of salvage therapies at a time when they may be more likely to be effective.

Following the Radical Prostatectomy

Radical prostatectomy results, ideally, in the complete extirpation of all malignant and benign prostatic tissue. The serum PSA should therefore fall to undetectable levels after surgery. This low level should, assuming a serum half-life of 2 to 3 days, be achieved within 21 days of surgery (seven half-lives will reduce the serum PSA to less than 1% of its original value). Although the possibility remains that a small residuum of prostatic tissue capable of producing PSA may be left by the surgeon, or that periurethral glands may have residual PSA-producing capabilities, a detectable PSA at any time after surgery is conventionally regarded as treatment failure. In favor of this interpretation is the observation that detectable PSA after surgery rarely remains static. There is almost invariably an upward progression, although the rate of rise varies greatly. The median doubling time following relapse after surgery is around 12 months, but the range is widely spread. Partin and colleagues at the Johns Hopkins Hospital observed 51 men with detectable PSA until they clinically failed before intervening (21). When the men with microscopic lymph node disease were excluded, the ratio of local to distant failure was approximately 1:1. This is important, as it suggests that up to one-half of surgical failures have the potential for curative salvage by prostatic fossa irradiation. Our ability to distinguish occult local failures from occult distant failures is further enhanced by studying the PSA level and its rate of rise after surgery. Ninety-four percent of the men who ultimately proved to have local failure had an undetectable PSA straight after surgery that rose one or more years later. This fits

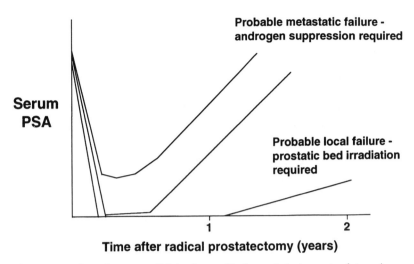

Fig. 4.1 *Using the serum PSA after radical prostatectomy to determine the most appropriate treatment if the PSA.*

neatly with the observation that radiation to the tumor bed infrequently cures men with a *persistently* detectable postoperative PSA (Fig. 4.1). Those with rates of PSA rise less than 1 ng/mL/yr are also far more likely to have locally persistent disease than distant, as are those with Gleason sums of 7 or less and no involvement of the seminal vesicles (22).

It has long been recognized that palpable local recurrences are well palliated by radiation but that these men are infrequently cured. This is presumably either because the tumor volume has become too large for radiation to sterilize or because allowing regrowth has also allowed a second chance for the tumor to metastasize. The use of PSA allows early salvage of local failures by radiation, perhaps increasing the potential for cure. In a number of recent reports it is clear that if salvage is to be successful, it must be offered very early, when the PSA is below 1–3 ng/mL. The case for close surveillance of surgically treated patients—with three monthly PSA assessments and prompt intervention in the case of those at particular risk for local failure—is thus strong. If follow-up appointments are spread too far apart, it would easily be possible for a patient to move from a curable to an incurable case between visits.

After Radical Radiation Therapy

The serum PSA cannot be used to detect failure quite so readily after radiation therapy as it can after surgery. This is because

1. the half-life of the PSA in the bloodstream is long, as cancer cells die slowly after potentially lethal irradiation when they next attempt to divide, and
2. the normal prostate gland remains in situ after radiation therapy and may continue to produce PSA.

There is general agreement that a progressively rising PSA constitutes failure, but it may be five or more years until this is seen. This does not allow for early assessment of the results of therapy or the early, and perhaps more successful, institution of salvage maneuvers. Many investigators have therefore sought an earlier PSA end point, examining the rate of PSA decline and the lowest level to which it declines (the nadir). Zagars and colleagues have suggested that unless the serum PSA falls to less than 2 ng/mL by 12 months, cure is unlikely (23). This, however, belies the common experience of the PSA's taking up to three years to decline to its nadir and has not found widespread favor. The notion of an "upper limit of normal" after radiation, much like the commonly accepted 4 ng/mL for untreated men with no prostate cancer, is appealing. Willett and associates showed that men who have received "incidental" prostatic irradiation as part of their treatment for bladder or rectal cancer have a median serum PSA of only 0.6 ng/mL, clearly demonstrating the ability of radiation to affect protein synthesis in the prostate (24) (Fig. 4.2). A similar phenomenon has been observed after irradiation of other organs, such as the pituitary for adenomas or the thyroid in Hodgkin's disease. Those men who are long-term disease-free survivors after radical high-dose radiation therapy for prostate cancer have a median PSA of 0.5 ng/mL or less. Seventy-eight percent have serum PSA levels below 1 ng/mL, and almost all are below 2 ng/mL. It does, therefore, seem that only those who achieve serum PSA nadirs below 1.0–1.5 ng/mL are likely to become long-term disease-free survivors.

When the PSA starts to climb again, the range of doubling times is wide, with a median around 12 months. The rate of rise may help

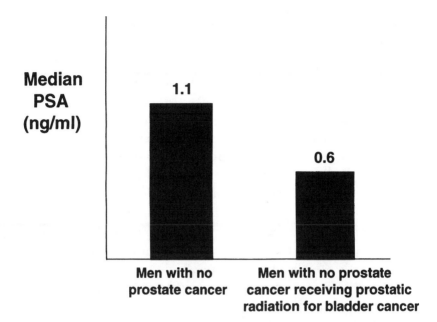

Fig. 4.2 *The effect of radiation on PSA production by the normal, healthy prostate gland. A study of men receiving incidental prostatic irradiation as part of their treatment for bladder or rectal cancer. (Reproduced by permission from Willett CG, Zietman AL, Shipley WU, Coen JJ. The effect of pelvic radiation therapy on the production of prostatic specific antigen. J Urol 1994;151:640–645.)*

to predict the interval until the development of clinical disease, perhaps influencing decisions about timing of androgen suppression. Hanks and colleagues have clearly shown that those with PSA doubling times of less than 3 months are likely to have clinical evidence of recurrent disease, usually metastases, within the year (25). These patients should probably start androgen suppression promptly to head off the inevitable symptomatic relapse. Those with a doubling time that exceeds a year may, if elderly or burdened with comorbidity, never see a clinical relapse in their lifetime. For these men, the weight gain and anemia of long-term androgen suppression may be quite unjustified and a policy of observation far more appropriate. Those with doubling times in between or with a very long life expectancy may, if highly motivated, be reevaluated for locally persistent disease by rebiopsy and be considered for early salvage prostatectomy. There is increasing evidence that, when performed early and by skilled hands, this salvage maneuver may be curative. One study from the Massachusetts General Hospital showed that fully 68% of men with palpably normal prostate glands after irradiation and a serum PSA in excess of 1 ng/mL had rebiopsies of their prostates that were positive for cancer (26).

It is of note that the doubling times of those relapsing after radiation or surgery are more rapid (median time, 12 months) than those seen in patients who are being observed and not actively treated (median, 24 to 48 months). This has been used as an argument against treatment by some, as it appears that debulking has somehow "revived up" the surviving cancer residuum. This argument is flawed for a number of reasons. First, those observed are selected for observation by virtue of their low potential for rapid progression. Second, the doubling time of those observed will eventually pick up speed if they are observed long enough. This is the classic "gompertzian" sigmoid pattern of tumor progression. Failures after treatment represent the same disease many years along and considerably further up the curve. The doubling time on failure reflects the initial tumor grade, showing that it is the biologic potential of the tumor, not the treatment, that is responsible for the pace of recurrence.

After Androgen Suppression

Androgen suppression is most commonly used in men with metastatic disease or in elderly men with symptomatic locally advanced disease. The duration of response has a median of two to three years, and once clinical progression has occurred, death usually follows within 12 to 18 months. The time to death is a little longer in men treated for locally advanced disease when compared with those with metastases.

Following the institution of hormonal ablative therapy, it is anticipated that the PSA will decrease. This is presumably as a result of two phenomena. The first is cell death resulting from androgen ablation. The other is a decrease in the expression of PSA from residual prostate cancer cells. This decreased expression occurs as a result of the fact that the PSA gene is under androgen control. Thus, the decrease in PSA following androgen deprivation does not clearly correlate with the degree of cell kill.

A correlation between the rate of fall of PSA and progression-free survival has not been proven. Many studies, however, have correlated the nadir PSA achieved and freedom from progression; the lower the level of PSA achieved, the longer the likelihood of progression-free survival.

A rise in the PSA is the earliest and most sensitive indicator of relapse after hormonal ablation. For patients with hormone-refractory prostate cancer, the interpretation of the PSA can be problematic. The interpretation that a rise in the PSA during this phase indicates progression of disease is widely accepted, although the clinical implications of a stable or decreasing PSA are more uncertain. Part of this difficulty in interpretation is due to the biologic fluctuation of the PSA at higher values. In addition, factors other than just tumor volume may in fact be contributing to serum levels of PSA. Nonetheless, the PSA has been used as a marker of tumor response in patients with hormone-refractory prostate cancer. Although the optimal level of decline of PSA is still somewhat debated, a PSA decline of more than 50% does correlate with an improved survival. However, one should be cautious about the overinterpretation of PSA responses in this setting.

As PSA gives advance warning of impending clinical failure, expensive and potentially toxic therapies, such as anti-androgens, may be promptly discontinued if ineffective. In the future, monitoring of PSA will allow earlier institution of more effective second-line therapies than are currently available—for example, growth factor antagonists or gene therapy. As PSA failure may precede death by 18 to 27 months, it may also be used as a surrogate for cancer-specific death, allowing the early analysis of trials of new agents for advanced disease.

■ PSA—FUTURE DIRECTIONS

Free Versus Bound PSA

Serum PSA circulates in two fractions: a free, unbound form and a bound form complexed to one of two serum protease inhibitors, $\alpha 1$ antichymotrypsin (ACT) or $\alpha 2$ macroglobulin (27). Recent reports have indicated that a greater proportion of serum PSA is complexed to ACT in prostate cancer than in BPH (28). Further studies have confirmed that the proportion of free PSA was lower in patients with prostate cancer that with BPH (29). Therefore, in the future, the free versus ACT bound serum PSA ratio may serve to identify patients who have prostate cancer more accurately than by using total PSA alone.

RT-PCR (Reverse Transcriptase Polymerase Chain Reaction) for PSA

PT-PCR for PSA utilizes molecular biological techniques that can identify small numbers of prostate cells in the peripheral circulation. The value of this test is that it is potentially far more sensitive than any presently available staging technique for prostate cancer, and it has the possibility of distinguishing patients with localized disease from systemic disease prior to therapy. The assay identifies PSA-synthesizing cells from reverse transcribed in RNA extracted from peripheral blood lymphocytes. An RT-PCR assay for PSA can recognize one PSA expressing cell diluted in 100,000 lymphocytes.

Although preliminary experience with RT-PCR has been encouraging (30–32), at the present time it is still considered investigational. Further work needs to be done to standardize the molecular techniques used among laboratories and to define the precise role of RT-PCR in distinguishing localized from metastatic disease.

Editorial Comment

Intelligent use of prostate-specific antigen has become an invaluable tool for the management of patients with prostate cancer. Potentially, PSA now plays a major role in diagnosis, assessment of disease extent, prognosis, selection of therapy, and monitoring response to therapy. When used in conjunction with other parameters such as Gleason grading, the accuracy of PSA for determining disease extent of prognosis may increase. In the future, newer tools, such as free versus bound PSA or RT-PCR, may improve diagnosis or assessment of disease extent even more.

Nevertheless, PSA levels may be misleading and misused. PSA is a marker for prostate epithelium not prostatic cancer. Many—in fact, most—patients who have an elevated PSA do not have prostate cancer. Although the level of PSA elevation may correlate with disease extent and prognosis, many patients with significant PSA elevation can be cured by aggressive local treatment. At the present time, determination of PSA alone should rarely be used either to promote or to rule out specific treatment recommendations for the individual patient.

PSA can also be used as a histochemical marker to diagnose anaplastic cancer cells of prostate origin. Used in this manner, it may be crucial in definitely diagnosing patients with adenocarcinoma of an "unknown" primary, and lead to the institution of appropriate therapy.

■ **REFERENCES**

1. Hara M, Inorre T, Fukuyama T. Some physico-chemical characteristics of gamma-seminoprotein, an antigenic component specific for human seminal plasma. Jpn J Legal Med 1971;5:322.
2. Wang MC, Valenzuela LA, Murphy GP, Chu TM. Purification of a human prostate specific antigen. Invest Urol 1979;17(2):159.
3. Lilja H, Laurell CB. Liquefaction of coagulated human semen. Scand J Clin Lab Invest 1984;44:447.
4. Oesterling JE. Prostate specific antigen: a critical assessment of the most useful tumor marker for adenocarcinoma of the prostate. J Urol 1991;145:907.
5. Ellis WJ, Brawer MK. PSA in benign prostatic hyperplasia and prostatic intraepithelial neoplasia. Urol Clin North America 1993;20(4):621.
6. Carter HB, Pearson JD. PSA velocity for the diagnosis of early prostate cancer. Urol Clin North Amer 1993;20(4):665.
7. Carter HB, Pearson JD, Metter JS, Brant LJ, Chan DW, Andres R, Fozard JL, Walsh PC. Longitudinal evaluation of prostate specific antigen levels in men with and without prostate disease. JAMA 1992;267:2215.
8. Seaman E, Whang M, Olsson CA, Katz A, Cooner WH, Benson MC. PSA density: role in patient evaluation and management. Urol Clin North Amer 1993;20(4):653–663.
9. Benson MC, Whang IS, Olsson CA, McMahon DJ, Cooner WH. The use of prostate specific antigen density to enhance the predictive value of intermediate levels of serum prostate specific antigen. J Urol 1992;147(3pt.2)817.
10. Brawer MK, Aramburu EAG, Chen GL, Preston SD, Ellis WJ. The inability of PSA index to enhance the predictive value of PSA in the diagnosis of prostatic carcinoma. J Urol 1993;150:369.
11. Oesterling JE, Jacobsen SJ, Chute CG, Guess HA, Girman CJ, Panser

LA, Lieber MM. Serum prostate specific antigen in a community based population of healthy men. Establishment of age specific reference ranges. JAMA 1993;270(7):860.

12. Prestigiacomo AF, Stamey TA. A comparison of 4 ultrasensitive prostate specific antigen assays for early detection of residual cancer after radical prostatectomy. J Urol 1994;152:1525.

13. Partin AW, Yoo J, Carter HB, et al. Use of prostate specific antigen, clinical stage, and Gleason score to predict pathological stage in men with localized prostate cancer. J Urol 1993;150:110–114.

14. Zietman AL, Coen JJ, Shipley WU, Efird J. Radical radiation therapy in the management of prostatic adenocarcinoma: the initial PSA value as a predictor of treatment outcome. J Urol 1994;151:640–645.

15. Zietman AL, Edelstein RA, Coen JJ, et al. Radical prostatectomy for adenocarcinoma of the prostate: the influence of pre-operative and pathologic findings on biochemical disease-free outcome. Urology 1994;43:828–833.

16. Schellhammer PF, El-Mahdi AM, Wright GL, et al. Prostate-specific antigen to determine progression-free survival after radiation therapy for localized carcinoma of prostate. Urology 1993;42:13–20.

17. Pisansky TM, Cha SS, Earle JD, et al. Prostate-specific antigen as a pretherapy prognostic factor in patients treated with radiation therapy for clinically localized prostate cancer. J Clin Oncol 1993;11: 2158–2165.

18. Leibel SA, Zelefsky MJ, Kutcher GJ, et al. Three-dimensional conformal radiation therapy in localized carcinoma of the prostate: interim report of a phase I dose-escalation study. J Urol 1994;152:1792–1798.

19. Blasko JC, Grimm PD, Ragde H. Brachytherapy and organ preservation in the management of carcinoma of the prostate. Semin Radiat Oncol 1993;3:240–249.

20. Pilepich MV, Krall JM, Al-Sarraf M, et al. Androgen deprivation with radiation therapy alone for locally advanced prostatic carcinoma: a randomized comparative trial of the Radiation Therapy Oncology Group. Urology 1995;45:616–623.

21. Partin AW, Pound CR, Pearson JD, et al. Evaluation of serum prostate specific antigen velocity after radical prostatectomy to distinguish local recurrence from distant metastases. Urology 1994;43:649–659.

22. McCarthy JF, Catalona WJ, Hudson MA. Effect of radiation therapy on detectable serum prostate specific antigen levels following radical prostatectomy: early versus delayed treatment. J Urol 1994;151:1575–1578.

23. Zagars GK. Serum PSA as a marker for patients undergoing definitive radiation therapy. Urol Clin North Am 1993;20:737–747.

24. Willett CG, Zietman AL, Shipley WU, Coen JJ. The effect of pelvic radiation therapy on the production of prostatic specific antigen. J Urol 1994;151:1579–1581.

25. Hanks GE, D'Amico A, Epstein BE, Schultheiss TE. Prostate-specific antigen doubling times in patients with prostate cancer: a potentially useful reflection of tumor doubling time. Int J Radiat Oncol Biol Phys 1993;27:125–127.

26. Dugan T, Shipley W, Young R, et al. Biopsy after external beam radiation therapy for adenocarcinoma of the prostate: correlation with original histologic grade and current PSA levels. J Urol 1991;146:1313.

27. Lilja H. Significance of different molecular forms of serum PSA. Urol Clin North America 1993;20(4):681.

28. Stenman VH, Leinonen J, Alfthan H, Rannikko S, Tuhkanen K, Alfthan O. A complex between prostate specific antigen and α1-antichymotrypsin is a major form of prostate specific antigen in serum of patients with prostatic cancer: Assay of the complex improves clinical sensitivity for cancer. Cancer Res 1991;51:222.

29. Christensson A, Bjork T, Nilsson O, Dohlen U, Matidainen MT, Cockett AT, Abrahamsson PA, Lilja H. Serum prostate specific antigen completed to alph 1-antichymotrypsin as an indicator of prostate cancer. J Urol 1993;150(1):100.

30. Katz AE, Olsson CA, Raffo AJ, Cama C, Perlman H, Seaman E, O'Toole KM, McMahon D, Benson MC, Buttyan R. Molecular staging of prostate cancer with the use of an enhanced reverse transcriptase PCR assay. Urology 1994;43(6):765.

31. Cama C, Olsson CA, Raffo AJ, Perlman H, Buttyan R, O'Toole K, McMahon D, Benson MC, Katz AE. Molecular staging of prostate cancer II. A comparison of the application of an enhanced reverse transcriptase polymerase chain reaction assay for prostate specific antigen versus prostate specific membrane antigen. J Urol 1995;153:1373.

32. Seiden MV, Kantoff PW, Krithivas D, Propert K, Bryant M, Haltom E, Gaynes L, Kaplan I, Bubley G, DeWolf W, et al. Detection of circulating tumor cells in men with localized prostate cancer. J Clin Oncol 1994;12(12):2634.

Observation

▼   ▼   ▼   ▼   ▼   ▼   ▼   ▼

William DeWolf
Marc B. Garnick
C. Norman Coleman

5

PROSTATE cancer appears to be a normal phenomenon of aging. That is to say, as men grow older, the *microscopic* incidence of prostate cancer becomes significant. This information is not new. For example, in 1954 Franks examined 210 men who had died of unknown causes and for whom a coroner's examination was required to establish the cause of death (1). Histologic assessment of prostatic disease was evaluated, with whole mount sections taken at 4mm intervals; 38% of these men had invasive prostate cancer. In fact, among the 17 men in their eighth decade of life, the incidence was 67%. Balanced against this high incidence, however, is the fact that only 8% of men develop clinically apparent prostate cancer (i.e., clinical stages T1b, T2, T3, and T4) that affects the quality of their life (2). Furthermore, only 3% of American men die of this disease (3). This enormous disparity between the very high incidence and the relatively low death rate, which, interestingly, applies only to prostate cancer, forms the basis for this chapter. How can issues related to slow growth rate, late-onset incidence, improved diagnostics, and treatment technology be integrated into a meaningful treatment algorithm such that clinically "insignificant" tumors will not be treated? These factors will be unraveled by first looking at what is known about the natural history of prostate cancer with subsequent comment on difficulties of data analysis and observation. To follow will be an analysis of what is known regarding our ability to separate "good" tumors from "bad" tumors, in an attempt to spare patients the morbidity of treatment for "insignificant" disease.

■ NATURAL HISTORY OF PROSTATE CANCER

How to Interpret the Literature

Prostate cancer, while indolent, is not a benign disease. Untreated patients will progress over time, with the rate of progression dependent on the tumor characteristics. Since death from all causes increases over time, the decision to diagnose, observe, or treat is dependent on the natural history of the particular patient, and is related to age and comorbid problems. For the overall U.S. male population, the life expectancies (the average years of life remaining) for individuals at the given ages are: 65—16 years; 70—12 years; 75—9 years; 80—7 years; and 85—5 years (4).

The first analysis to be made is the risk of death for the individual patient, based on his age and general state of health. This risk is then compared with the risk of progression of the prostate cancer. Three numbers should be estimated: 1) the risk of local disease progression such that treatment will be required for symptomatic relief; 2) the risk of developing debility from the disease and its treatment (debility can result from symptoms due to local progression, metastatic disease, or the side effects of systemic or local therapy); and 3) the risk of dying from prostate cancer. Unfortunately, precise numbers for each of these risks are difficult to ascertain.

Another factor to consider is that *apparent* improved survival from early detection by screening and subsequent treatment may be due to *lead time* and *length time bias* (5). Lead time bias assumes that the disease will run its course. With an earlier diagnosis, however, the survival time will appear to be improved simply because the diagnosis was made at an earlier time in the patient's life. Length time bias relates to the rate of disease progression. Compared with a rapidly growing and more aggressive cancer, the more slowly growing tumors (which are discovered earlier) are more likely to have a longer "preclinical" phase—that is, a phase in which a screening test may diagnose the cancer but before it would have become a symptomatic problem (5). Due to their longer preclinical phase, less aggressive tumors are more likely to be picked up by routine screening than more aggressive tumors, so it can be argued that the majority of tumors caught in a screening net are those that were less likely to be a clinical problem. However, it could also be argued that these less aggressive cancers are the ones with a lower metastatic potential and are more likely to be cured by local therapy. Screening data indicate that most cancers picked up on initial screening (so-called prevalent cases) look like cancers that might be clinically significant, with approximately one-fourth to one-third having already extended beyond the capsule of the gland (6,7).

The most appropriate and useful data addressing the benefits of treatment are obtained from large randomized trials, in which the lead and length time biases are equally distributed. Randomized trials are difficult to conduct due to limited participation by patients and physicians (8,9). Patients entered in randomized trials are not necessarily representative of the general population (10), and even when such trials are conducted, the results are applicable only to those patients who have characteristics similar to those in the randomized trials. As will be discussed below, this is particularly important in observation trials, as many of them are conducted with very selected populations, based on clinical or pathologic status, or both.

Even more difficult to use in practice are treatment results from single-institution series, due to the often unknown patient selection bias for a particular series. Results that include all patients seen in an institution would be most representative of the "real world"; however, in most published series only a fraction of the patients seen are included. Lastly, the handling of patients who are lost to follow-up or who die of "other causes" (intercurrent death) is important in interpreting the results of a study. Such patients are often censored from the disease-progression curve; that is, it is assumed that they are doing well at the time they were lost to follow-up. This would lead to an underestimation of the true risk of disease recurrence. More recently, many statisticians have insisted that patients lost to follow-up should be considered as having failed, which might lead to an overestimation of disease recurrence. In making heads or tails of the literature, it is important that the reader be aware of the analytical technique that has been used.

Making the Decision

Clinical decisions must be made without all the necessary information at hand. What is known about the natural history of prostate cancer comes inferentially from historical pathologic reviews and from a limited number of observation trials. Perhaps the most important bias involved is that of patient preference. Patients' decisions are influenced by the media, personal experience, and the opinion of their physicians.

The important message of this chapter is that *prostate cancer is not a benign entity, and if left untreated it will progress.* The rate of progression may be extraordinarily low in very favorable settings and surprisingly rapid in others. The prognostic factors, discussed elsewhere in this book, relate to the inherent tumor biology. The questions of when to treat and which treatment to use have not been answered with certainty. But if curative therapy is intended, it is important to remember that the probability of cure decreases with time. Ideally, one would apply a very effective local treatment just before the cancer develops resistance and metastatic properties. In the future, but certainly not now, it may be possible to evaluate these molecular and cellular properties in the decision-making process.

Natural Progression of Prostate Cancer

The increasing incidence of prostate cancer over time has led investigators to suggest that many of the cancers are present for years or even decades (11). The time lag between rise in incidence rate and mortality rate further suggests that, on average, there is a long delay, perhaps one to two decades, between when a cancer can be diagnosed and when it can be fatal (12). Such a statistic belies the potential morbidity of the cancer, however, since patients will be under treatment for some time during this interval and may well have substantial symptoms from local or systemic disease.

The progression rate of patients who have undergone initial observation indicates that many patients will require treatment within 5 to 10 years. Reports by Blute and colleagues (13) and Stillwell and colleagues (14) on patients with stage T1 disease (nonpalpable and confined to the prostate) indicate that about 40% of patients will have progressed within the first decade, with the progression rate being somewhat greater for those with more extensive disease. For patients with cancer detected by transurethral resection of the prostate (TURP), the rate of progression can be estimated from their Gleason score and the percentage of tissue involved with cancer. Lowe and

Barry estimated the probability of disease progression within 5 years for a number of clinical scenarios. For patients with Gleason scores (on a scale of 2 to 10) of 4 or lower, and less than 5% of the tissue involved with tumor, the 5-year progression rate ranges to 5% to 10%. For those with a Gleason score of 5 or 6, the progression rate ranges to 30% to 60%, depending on the extent of involvement. Patients with more than 5% of tissue involved had a progression rate in excess of 50%. For those with Gleason scores of 7 to 9, the rate of progression was approximately 50% for those with less than 5% involvement and approximately 80% for those with more extensive disease (15).

For the primary care doctor, it must be emphasized that the extent of disease found at the time of TURP might not be an adequate predictor of disease progression. Due to the multifocal nature of the disease and its predilection for location in the peripheral zone rather than the transitional zone (which is what is removed at the TURP), the cancer not sampled by the TURP may be the greater potential problem (16). This would necessitate a more complete workup, including imaging studies and additional biopsies.

The rate of local progression is higher for patients with palpable cancer (clinical stage T2). Whitmore and associates (17) reported on the results of expectant management of patients with stage T2 disease, most of whom had well or moderately well differentiated tumors. Local progression occurred in 50% of the patients by 5 years and in about 80% of patients by 10 years. At 10 years, about 30% of the patients had distant progression.

Prostate cancer is not a benign disease, and over time the risk of dying of prostate cancer will increase. Lerner and colleagues studied 360 patients with localized prostate cancer (stages T1b, T2, T3) who underwent staging pelvic lymphadenectomy and radiation therapy, including interstitial implant and external beam. The risk of dying of prostate cancer was 8% ± 3% (±2 standard errors) at 5 years and 30% ± 7% at 10 years, while the risk of death from all causes (including prostate cancer) was 16% ± 4% at 5 years and 46% ± 7% at 10 years (18). This illustrates that, over time, more prostate cancer patients die of prostate cancer than other causes, which is particularly true with younger patients, who have a lower risk of intercurrent death (11). This general observation has been interpreted to mean that patients expected to have a prolonged survival, perhaps 10 years or more, can benefit from radical treatment (19–21).

Theoretical Concerns

Leaving the toxicity of treatment aside for the moment, when one approaches the concept of observation with an individual patient who has clinically localized disease, an important assumption is made that there is little risk of deferring local treatment. This may be a valid statement if there is already micrometastatic disease or if the tumor will remain localized and still be amenable to curative treatment should the need exist. A theoretical risk, however, and a component of observation, is whether the progression of the tumor will be linear over an extended period of time. Molecular biologic studies have recently demonstrated the presence of a "mutator phenotype" (22–24). Once acquired, the cell may have a propensity to mutate faster, so that mutations may accumulate rapidly once the phenotype is present. Although the role of such mutations has yet to be determined in prostate cancer, these theoretical issues should be considered. Among the emotional issues that often lead a patient to accept treatment is the *uncertainty* as to the detrimental effect of delayed therapy.

With unknown benefits of treatment and undefined risks of an initial course of observation, the issue of toxicity then becomes quite important. Reducing the morbidity of local treatment is, perhaps, as important an issue as increasing the efficacy of the treatment. The benefits and risks of the various treatment options for incidental cancers have been reviewed (25) and are discussed further elsewhere in this book.

In the next section, the major observation trials will be discussed in some detail, so that the primary physician will have sufficient information when advising patients and answering their questions regarding the selection of treatment versus observation.

■ WATCHFUL WAITING

What Is Watchful Waiting?

The subject of "watchful waiting" is particularly problematic. In everyday terminology, watchful waiting has come to mean the absence of any active treatment intervention in the management of patients with prostate cancer. Generally, some aspects of disease activity will trigger active intervention. Disease activity may be suspected by a determination of rising PSA or a worsening of physical abnormalities on examination of the prostate gland in the case of patients with localized disease. For patients with advanced disease, disease activity may mean the worsening of bone scan abnormalities or the development of symptoms secondary to worsening metastatic disease.

The thinking that prostate cancer is a disease of an aging population that may not require active treatment—if, for example, it is diagnosed in an elderly patient with significant comorbid diseases and limited life expectancy—is entirely appropriate, and should often be encouraged. It is the concept of watchful waiting as currently being applied to younger patients that needs to be carefully analyzed, for it is here that major mistakes can be made.

The Data Against Treatment

Three recent papers are often cited as evidence against invasive treatment (20,26,27). The first, entitled "High 10-Year Survival Rate in Patients with Early, Untreated Prostatic Cancer," written by Johansson and colleagues in Sweden (26), evaluated 223 patients with T0–2, NX, M0 disease. No definitive therapy after the initial diagnosis of prostate cancer was provided. In other words, no specific treatment was administered until symptoms requiring intervention or metastatic disease developed, at which time specific treatment was given. Over a mean follow-up of 123 months, the 10-year disease-specific survival was 86.8%, with a confidence interval of 81 to 165 months. Because the survival was comparable to a cohort of patients who would have met the criteria for receiving a radical prostatectomy, the authors concluded that evaluation of any local or systemic therapy for early prostate cancer must use untreated controls for comparison.

This article received much attention and provided a basis for advocating a policy of watchful waiting for patients with prostate cancer (28–30). Moreover, the article reinforced the teachings in medical school that prostate cancer is a disease that one dies *with* rather than *of*. While this approach is appropriate in patients who are elderly or who have competing causes of comorbid disease, the application of principles dictating nonintervention may have been inappropriately interpreted to apply to a younger patient population than those for whom it was not intended.

Critical analysis of the Johannson article deserves attention and will reveal flaws in the conclusions. Of the 223 patients who were followed, the cancer progressed in 76 patients during the course of the study. Fifty of these were found to have local extension, and 26 had metastatic spread. Of 152 patients who were felt to be "without signs of progression," 30 developed mild to moderate local problems, presumably due to local extension, requiring 14 to undergo a transurethral resection. The authors do not indicate whether cancer was found in any of the transurethral resection specimens. Moreover, in calculating the death rate in this untreated population, there were 105 patients who died from causes other than prostate cancer. Included were 3 patients who developed metastatic disease who were treated with estrogen therapy—yet these men were scored as deaths due to causes other than prostate cancer.

The criteria for patient selection in this Swedish study also deserves comment. For two years of the study, only patients with grade I, well-differentiated lesions were included. Between the years of 1979 and 1984, patients who were less than 75 years old were placed on a randomized treatment program assigning them to receive either radiation treatments or no treatment. Only those randomized to no treatment were also included in the current analysis. Patients more than 75 years old were not routinely treated, and those patients were also included in the study. Thus this was not a consecutively enrolled patient population but a highly biased, nonsequential group of patients, many of whom were elderly and had low-grade tumors, and it was clearly not representative of the patient in the United States who is younger and may have a more virulent tumor. Yet the message that has mistakenly gotten across to the thousands of men in the United

States is that a policy of watchful waiting is an acceptable treatment option. (The different outcomes experienced by this Swedish population of patients will be contrasted momentarily to a similarly staged population of patients treated some years earlier as part of the Veterans Administration Cooperative Urological Research Group Studies.)

A second article, entitled "A Decision Analysis of Alternative Treatment Strategies for Clinically Localized Prostate Cancer" (the Prostate Patient Outcomes Research Team or PPORT study) has become a focal point for keeping the debate alive regarding no-treatment policies (27). The findings of the authors of this report support watchful waiting. Among the conclusions of this study were the following: for well-differentiated tumors, treatment at best offers limited benefit—and may result in harm. For moderately and poorly differentiated tumors in patients 60 to 65 years old, treatment benefits could result from either radical prostatectomy or radiation therapy, compared with watchful waiting. Additionally, invasive treatment of clinically localized prostate cancer appeared to be harmful for patients older than 70 years.

In arriving at these conclusions, the authors chose from selected literature references various complication rates resulting from treatment programs. Mathematical determinations of rates of developing metastatic cancer in series with watchful waiting as a policy were calculated and incorporated into the decision analysis paradigm.

The widespread medical and lay coverage that accompanied this research was unprecedented. From headlines in the *Wall Street Journal* to articles in nearly every local daily newspaper, the chilling conclusion from these findings was that perhaps entirely too much treatment and treatment-related suffering was being advocated and delivered to patients.

Careful analyses of the PPORT data indicate many flaws. One major flaw relates to the selection of patients for determination of rates of developing metastatic disease. Five citations (31–35) were selected and incorporated into the mathematical model for determining rates of development of metastatic disease "based on several large studies of patients managed with 'watchful waiting' alone." Implicit in the methods section of the report was the assumption that these patients were diagnosed with prostate cancer and did not receive any active intervention until the development of symptoms. This statement, whether implicitly or explicitly accepted, is *frankly incorrect*. For example, two studies from which metastatic progression rates were selected, included patients with clinically localized cancer who did not receive radical prostatectomy but instead received early hormonal treatment (35) or open prostatectomy (34). The hormonally treated patients were part of the so-called focal carcinoma study (35) in which patients with stage 1 (current stage A or T1) were thought to be too ill or too old, or they refused radical prostatectomy. However, contrary to the statement in the PPORT study, these patients did not receive watchful waiting, but rather were randomized to receive treatment with diethylstilbestrol, orchiectomy plus placebo, orchiectomy plus diethylstilbestrol, or placebo alone (35). Thus, three-quarters, of the patients received active, systemic therapy for their early localized prostate cancer, not watchful waiting as implied by both the media and the report's authors.

Early systemic treatment for prostate cancer is an important issue that has an impact on the "natural history" of the disease, especially in a comparative analysis between these studies. In the focal carcinoma study of 148 patients (most of whom received hormonal therapy), there were 72 deaths during the five years of follow-up (35). It was remarkable that no patients during this time died from prostate cancer! In addition, only 10 of the 148 patients (6.7%) experienced progressive cancer. This is compared with the 34% to 49% progressive cancer rate in the Swedish study, although the focal carcinoma study patients were followed for a shorter length of time. The effects of treatment on the prostate gland were noteworthy. Of 22 patients on whom an autopsy was performed, residual cancer was found in only 1. Yet if one reads the PPORT study, none of this information is described. Any analysis utilizing patient rates of developing metastatic cancer from the focal carcinoma study and claiming successful treatment results from watchful waiting represents a misinterpretation of these earlier reports.

Additional problems with the PPORT study relate to the inclusion of only sexually active patients in the decision analysis. That these patients will have a markedly impaired quality of life following treatment that may affect their potency is understandable, but this does not adequately reflect the more typical population in whom treatment decisions are based not on maintenance of sexual function but rather on desire for survival. Additional criticisms have been listed against the methods of data collection and analysis (36).

A third publication, entitled "Results of Conservative Management of Clinically Localized Prostate Cancer" by Chodak and associates (20), was recently published and suffers from many of the same methodologic problems as the previous citations, mainly because the analysis included the same patient populations supporting a watchful waiting policy. Yet, again, the survival figures resulting from watchful waiting for the patient with a moderately or poorly differentiated cancer are dismal and demand novel and improved methods—not a nonintervention policy.

Finally, the overall concept of "noncurative" treatment (which technically is not the same as watchful waiting), is perhaps best understood by looking at a report by Aus, who performed a retrospective analysis of 536 patients with known diagnoses of prostate cancer who died in Göteborg, Sweden, between the years 1988 and 1990 (37). He found that the median cancer-specific survival time for well-differentiated or low-stage tumors (T2a) was approximately 15 years. However, this long survival was tempered by age at diagnosis. For example, of patients who were diagnosed with prostate cancer before the age of 55, 100% eventually died from the disease (Table 5.1).

■ CAN STAGING DISTINGUISH "GOOD" TUMORS FROM "BAD" TUMORS?

As the controversies and issues regarding the treatment of prostate cancer unfold, one question is repeatedly asked, and if it were answered, most of the problems regarding treatment would be solved. The question is: Of all the tumors present, which ones need be treated? What type of tumor will the patient die *with*, and what type of tumor will the patient die *of*? Unfortunately there is no biochemical or molecular marker that will provide us with such an answer. However, the presence (or absence) of certain physical features, plus consideration of age, will allow us to make an educated guess as to which tumors may be watched and which might pose a

Table 5.1 *Prostate Cancer Death Rate According to Age at Diagnosis*

Age at Diagnosis (yr)	Deaths from Prostate Cancer (%)
<55	100
60	75
65	70
70	60
75	55
80	45
>85	25

SOURCE: Aus G. Prostate cancer: mortality and morbidity after non-curative treatment with aspects on diagnosis and treatment. Scand J Urol Nephrol Suppl 1994;167:1–41.

threat to the patient's life. This information will have its greatest value to the older population, which will be balancing a naturally limited life expectancy against a possibly slow-growing tumor. Younger patients with a much longer life expectancy will benefit less from this information.

Tumor Volume

One of the most important features of prostate cancer, as well as other malignancies, is that the capacity of a tumor to metastasize is, in general, a function of its volume (38). In theory, prostate cancers may evolve from differentiated to poorly differentiated tumors with time; and during this time of cancer growth, size may be the best "yardstick" for measuring biologic potential. In perhaps the best and earliest study, Stamey performed morphometric reconstructions of 68 consecutive radical prostatectomies, revealing a strong interrelation between volume, extent of complete capsular penetration, microscopic seminal vesicle and lymph node invasion, and histologic differentiation (39). For example, at a tumor volume of less than 3.0 cc, only 6 of 34 prostates (18%) showed capsular penetration, compared with 28 of 34 (82%) that had tumors greater than 3.0 cc. Seminal vesicle invasion occurred in 1 of 34 tumors of less than 3.0 cc, and in 15 of 34 tumors greater than 3.0 cc. Finally, all 6 patients with metastases to lymph nodes—2 with early postoperative bone metastases and 4 or 5 with reappearance of detectable bone metastases—had cancer volumes of greater than 4.0 cc.

It is therefore apparent that a tumor size of 3 to 4 cc is a critical limit with regard to biologic containment to the prostate; but then, is there a smaller size that tells us that a tumor is so small that *treatment* can be deferred? This is perhaps the most important question. The most conservative estimate for a clinically insignificant tumor is 0.2 cc. This is based on several "circumstantial" pieces of evidence. For example, of 21 radical prostatectomy specimens with a tumor volume less than 0.2 cc, none demonstrated capsular penetration and none demonstrated disease progression as defined by measurable postoperative PSA levels (mean follow-up, five years) (40,41). Likewise, most incidentally discovered prostate cancers, either at autopsy or by specimen examination after cystoprostatectomy with unsuspected prostate cancer, are usually less than 0.2 cc in size (42). In another series of 139 men undergoing cystoprostatectomy for bladder cancer, none of whom was suspected of having prostate cancer, 55 were found to have cancer of the prostate (43). Fifty percent of those individuals had a tumor volume of less than 0.05 cc, and most of them measured 3 to 4 mm when observed in the plane of greatest dimension under the microscope. Additional studies support the correlation between tumor size and invasiveness by indicating that tumors of less than 0.1 cc never had seminal vesicle invasion, and only 1 of 56 autopsy cancers less than 0.46 cc had complete capsular penetration, compared with 17 of 33 tumors greater than 0.46 cc (38,44). If we consider that "insignificant" lesions are either 0.2 cc or 0.5 cc, and look at prostates removed at surgery, an interesting observation may be made (45). If T1c lesions are compared with T2 lesions, 16% versus 2% are insignificant if 0.2 cc is the cutoff, and 26% versus 5% are insignificant if 0.5 cc is the cutoff (Table 5.2). In general, these "insignificant" lesions occur only with T1c tumors (or T1a tumors, but they are becoming rare) and not in T2 lesions; if a lesion is palpable, it is most likely "significant." Interestingly, the smallest cancer detected by digital rectal exam was 0.2 cc, which, if

Table 5.2 *Association of stage and "insignificant disease according to tumor volume*

| Preoperative Stage | Tumors Found to Be Insignificant | |
	Volume <0.2 cc*	*Volume <0.5 cc**
T1a	33%	25%
T1c	16%	10%
T2	2%	3%

*From radical prostatectomy specimens.

SOURCE: Epstein J, Walsh P, Carmichael M, Brendler C. Pathologic and clinical findings to predict tumor extent in nonpalpable (stage T1c) prostate cancer. JAMA 1994;271:368–374.

present in the shape of a sphere, would measure 0.7 cm in diameter (46). Remember that if the cancer is found on the side opposite a *benign* nodule, then the cancer must be considered T1c rather than T2 (see Chapter 3).

Grade

Several studies have shown that, in addition to the volume of a cancer, the Gleason grade is an important determinant in differentiating "significant" from insignificant cancer (39,43,47). (See Chapter 2 for an explanation of the Gleason grading system.) This is based on the simplistic and logical concept that patients with well and moderately differentiated tumors do far better than patients with poorly differentiated tumors (Gleason score 4 or 5, or Gleason sum 8 to 10). Grade has been shown to be an independent predictor of clinical progression even in Japan, where clinical disease is less prevalent (48). In general, a substantial amount of tumor of Gleason grade 4 or 5 is required for lymph node metastases (44). One important fact to remember, however, is that biopsies are not often able to predict the grade adequately, especially in identifying high-grade lesions. For example, in one series of 316 patients, there were 15 patients who, by radical prostatectomy, had high-grade lesions (Gleason sum 8 to 10).

Of these 15 patients, only 8 were correctly predicted by needle biopsy, giving a significant error rate. This, of course, represents one of the pitfalls of basing an algorithm on biopsy grade (49).

Is There a Way to Identify an "Insignificant" Cancer Using Tumor Volume and Grade?

In this section we will use the terms *significant* and *insignificant* to characterize tumors that have the volume and grade that are felt to be likely or unlikely to progress and be lethal.

For the most part, if a tumor is palpable, then it is larger than 0.2 cc in volume and is probably not insignificant. It is important to remember, however, that nodules are often nonmalignant and that cancer can be incidentally found elsewhere in the gland "by accident." Therefore, a patient with a nodule that is benign by biopsy may also have a malignant focus away from the nodule that could be insignificant. The best retrospective study looking at this problem evaluated 157 men who underwent radical retropubic prostatectomy for nonpalpable disease (45). Biopsies were done for either an abnormal or rising PSA, or an abnormal imaging study. Only 16% had insignificant tumors by a conservative measure (less than 0.2 cc), and another 10% by less stringent criteria (less than 0.5 cc). No single variable, including grade, PSA level, PSA density, transrectal ultrasound results, and age, adequately predicted insignificant tumor, with the negative predictive values being as low as 43%, 42%, and 33% for PSA level, PSA density greater than 0.1 ng/mL per gram of prostate tissue, and PSA density 0.15 ng/mL per gram, respectively.

A multivariate analysis, however, proved more informative. Using variables such as PSA less than 4.0, PSA density less than 0.1, Gleason scores less than 4, no core more than 50% involved, and fewer than three cores involved, the best model to predict significant cancer was a PSA density greater than 0.1 ng/mL per gram with any "bad" pathologic variable on needle biopsy of the prostate (Table 5.3). This model correctly identified 92% of advanced tumors. The problem, however, concerns the negative predictive value, which in this case signifies how often, when a preoperative clinical parameter predicted insignificant tumor, insignificant tumor was in fact found. In this case, the values never go above the mid-60% range (Table 5.3).

Table 5.3 *Clinical Predictors for Significant Disease*[†]

Preoperative Clinicopathologic Findings			Positive Predictive Value, %**	Negative Predictive Value, %**
PSA	*Pathology**	*PSA Density*		
<4 (and)	good			61
≥4 (or)	bad		89	
	good (and)	<0.1		63
	bad (or)	≥0.1	92	

*Bad pathologic findings include Gleason Score 4 or 5, or three or more core samples involved, or any core sample more than 50% involved. "Good" pathologic findings indicate the absence of all findings listed as "bad" pathologic findings.
**The positive predictive value defines how often, when a preoperative clinical parameter predicted significant tumor, there was actually significant tumor within the radical prostatectomy specimen. The negative predictive value defines how often, when a preoperative clinical parameter predicted insignificant tumor, insignificant tumor was in fact present.

[†] >0.2 cc

SOURCE: Epstein J, Walsh P, Carmichael M, Brendler C. Pathologic and clinical findings to predict tumor extent in nonpalpable (stage T1c) prostate cancer. JAMA 1994;271:368–374.

Importantly, this study showed several interesting things. First, if cancer can be found by needle biopsy, then it is usually significant, irrespective of any other criteria. That is to say, 84% of T1c lesions had volumes of greater than 0.2 cc. Second, if a tumor is palpable, then it generally is greater than 0.2 cc in volume and is, therefore, significant (Table 5.2). Third, nonpalpable tumors are particularly treacherous simply because one of the cancer-monitoring parameters—palpability—happens to be lost. The cause of the nonpalpability is usually not known, but several possibilities exist: for example, an anterior or central location of the tumor, BPH, or lack of tumor desmoplasia. Fourth, transrectal ultrasound was not predictive of tumor extent. Fifth, pathologic findings on needle biopsy helped predict significant lesions *but were not always correct.* For example, any one of three pathologic variables predicted significant disease: 1) any Gleason score 4 or 5; 2) three or more core samples with tumor involvement; and 3) any core with 50% or more tumor involvement. Importantly, favorable pathologic findings on needle biopsy did not guarantee favorable pathologic features in the excised prostate.

These principles have been confirmed in other series. In one series of 28 patients who had undergone radical prostatectomy and who had 3 mm or less of prostate cancer in only one core of at least six biopsies and a Gleason sum of not greater than 4/10, 16 had a cancer volume of 0.2 cc or less, and 7 had a volume of 0.2 to 0.5 cc (50). Several attempts have been made to construct formulas that will reliably predict volume of cancer; unfortunately, however, to date none is available that is satisfactory for the individual patient (51). In another study of 130 patients, correlating volume of cancer in the biopsy with volume of cancer in the radical prostatectomy specimen found there was a direct correlation. However, there was significant variability in prostate cancer volume for a given percentage of cancer in the biopsy specimen: i.e., the standard error of the estimate was 6.1 mL. In fact, of 13 patients with 5% or less cancer volume and a Gleason score less than 7 in the biopsy specimen, only 1 (8%) had a cancer volume smaller than 0.5 mL in the radical prostatectomy specimen (52). To make matters worse, rebiopsy is fraught with significant error and inconsistency, making uncertainty an integral part of correct prediction of significant disease (53).

Age

As previously noted, the impact of watchful waiting and the selection of patients who can safely be observed depends heavily on the lead time achieved by screening and the time between detection and death due to prostate cancer. Clinical prostate cancer has been shown to develop 6 to 10 years after serum PSA exceeds 4 ng/mL, which corresponds to a tumor volume of 1.0 cc and a diameter of 1.2 cm (54). This assumes a doubling time of 2 years. A tumor of 0.2 cc will require an additional 5 years to reach a size of 1.0 cc. Thus, men with insignificant prostate cancers of 0.2 cc are expected to develop clinically significant tumors in about 15 years, with a median survival beyond that time of about 3.6 years (55). Therefore, observation of insignificant disease is most likely to benefit patients whose life expectancy is about 15 years or less (see Table 5.1). Because the normal life expectancy of a person aged 65 is 15 years, the conclusion is that watchful waiting is appropriate only for patients thought to have insignificant disease who are above the age of 65 at the very least.

MRI

Attempts to stage prostate cancer by endorectal coil MR images, either by volume or by capsular penetration, have been reported, but without satisfactory results. For example, in one study of 30 patients, MRI identified only 41 of 85 lesions, or 48% (56). More important, of the peripheral zone lesions, which should be the easiest to identify by MRI, only 41 of 56 (73%) were identified; of these, the sizes of 16 (39%) were grossly over- or underestimated by at least 50%. In fairness to the study, of the 15 lesions in the peripheral zone not identified on MR images, 9 occurred in areas of hemorrhage. These findings, however, make it extremely unlikely that MRI technology, at least as currently used, is good enough to accurately assess a 0.2- to 0.5-cc lesion and track its size over time. Whether MR enhancement or MR-guided biopsies will alter the usefulness of endorectal MRI remains to be seen.

Ploidy

Thus far we have indicated that there are but a few objective markers of malignant potential of an individual focus of prostate cancer—that is, grade and volume of cancer. Another criterion that has been investigated is DNA ploidy, which has already been shown to correlate with recurrence and survival in multivariate analyses, in that diploid tumors tend to do much better than nondiploid tumors (57). The idea is that, as tumors grow, they develop genetic instability with a resultant increase in malignant potential. Indeed, tumor ploidy has been found to correlate with tumor volume. In one study, all tumors less than 0.02 cc in size were diploid (58). In that study, involving 63 cancers from 30 patients undergoing radical prostatectomy, the positive predictive value of nondiploidy in predicting a tumor to be greater than 0.2 or 0.5 cc in size was 86% and 82%, respectively. More important, the negative predictive value of diploidy in predicting a tumor to be less than either 0.2 or 0.5 cc in size was only 54% and 75%, respectively, which is probably not sufficient to bet that a tumor is

Table 5.4 *Some molecular markers currently under investigation to predict tumor behavior*

p53	EGFr end EGF
ras	IGF-1
c-myc	bcl-2
c-sis	bFGF
RB	androgen receptor
E Cadherin	telomerase
int-2	

insignificant. In general, there was significant association between tumor volume and ploidy, but there were frequent exceptions with nondiploid cell populations observed in several small cancer volumes as low as 0.03 cc. Furthermore, of 24 cancers less than 1 cc in volume, 8 were nondiploid and 3 had extracapsular extension. In general, these findings do not support the view that malignant potential is acquired in a predictable progressive manner totally related to cancer volume.

Molecular Markers

We have looked at conventional pathologic features of in situ prostate cancer in an attempt to characterize and differentiate between slow-growing insignificant cancers and those cancers that are significant and grow beyond the confines of the prostate. As expected, these relatively "gross" approaches will usually be correct, but will have an inherent error rate of about 20% to 25%. What is needed, quite logically, is an understanding of the molecular events that lead up to the metastatic capability so that these tumors can be monitored, giving the clinician an "early warning" system that would allow for the tumor to be removed or the cancer otherwise cured before it becomes harmful to the patient. As always, this assumes that the patient's life expectancy is long enough that a cure would prolong his life, an issue which should always be kept in mind when dealing with the older patient population. Unfortunately, at the present time there are no accepted molecular features of prostate cancer that allow us to predict tumor behavior *accurately*. Several markers, however, are under investigation (Table 5.4). Perhaps the best known is p53, a protein intimately involved in cell cycle regulation, apoptosis, and, perhaps, differentiation. In general, p53 mutations are considered rare in primary tumors and appear coincident with advanced disease, dedifferentiation, and androgen independence (59). The problem, however, is that these findings are not totally uniform, due, in fact, to the lack of uniform testing procedures (60,61).

■ **CONCLUSION**

How do we untangle this most significant puzzle facing the hundreds of thousands of men who will be diagnosed with prostate cancer in the next few years? Through the use of PSA-based screening programs, the identification of early and possibly highly curable prostate cancer is within our grasp (62,63). In many instances, watchful waiting for highly selected men is appropriate and should be encouraged. This is especially true for patients with lower grade tumors (i.e., Gleason sum 6 or less) and a life expectancy less than 10 years. If there were a reliable method to predict "low volume disease" accurately, then more men could be entered into this group. Unfortunately, such a method does not yet exist. To widely endorse watchful waiting, however, based on an incomplete understanding and analysis of the data, allowing many patients to miss a chance for cure, should not be recommended. This is especially true as there are no appropriate randomized prospective studies to support such a policy. *Patients need to be informed of this.* At a recent American Urological Association meeting, a prominent advocate of appropriate treatment practices reflected that the 70-year-old man with metastatic prostate cancer may have been, 20 years earlier, a 50-year-old man with a curable prostate cancer (64). A full discussion of the side effects of treatment must be encouraged, to allow the patient and the physician to make an informed treatment choice. The advances that are being made in surgical techniques, improved delivery and safety of radiation therapy, and improved understanding of both the timing and the types of hormonal therapy, combined with superior diagnostic methods to detect, treat, and cure more prostate cancers, should be enthusiastically embraced until definitive evidence against them is provided.

Editorial Comment

Although it is apparent that many patients with prostate cancer do not require treatment, the selection of such patients is complex. Clearly, generalizations such as "treatment is of no benefit to patients" is as problematic as "all patients should undergo aggressive local treatment." The authors of this chapter give an objective and scholarly appraisal of this complex area and caution us in the interpretation of retrospective case series, particularly those that have been published on observation.

The group of patients for whom observation is a reasonable treatment approach are those whose life expectancy is limited due to age or comorbidity. A reasonable rule of thumb, based on the best available data, is that patients whose age or comorbidity would lead to a life expectancy of less than 10 years may not need to undergo treatment. Such patients should probably not have undergone screening for prostate cancer in the first place. For patients at the other end of the spectrum—younger patients, those under 60, who are otherwise healthy—we recommend treatment because of the uncertain natural history of prostate cancer and the difficulties in following patients. For patients in between these two extremes it is most difficult to determine the best approach. For the otherwise healthy 60- to 70-year-old man, the hope is that tumor characteristics, including grade and volume, will guide therapy decisions. In general, we are hesitant to recommend observation if more than one core sample is involved or the Gleason score is greater than 6. For some patients with a Gleason score of 6 or less and just one positive core sample, observation should be part of the discussion, with a decision based on the risks and benefits.

■ REFERENCES

1. Franks LM. Latent carcinoma of the prostate. J Pathol 1954;68: 603–616.
2. Stamey TA, Freiha FS, McNeal JE, et al. Localized prostate cancer: relationship of tumor volume to clinical significance of prostate cancer. Cancer 1993;71:933–938.

3. Seidman H, Mushinski MH, Gelb SK, Silverberg E. Probabilities of eventually developing or dying of cancer. CA 1985;36:56.

4. Welch GH, Albertsen PC, Nease RF, et al. Estimating treatment benefits for the elderly: the effect of competing risks. Ann Intern Med 1996;124:577–584.

5. Black WC, Welch HG. Advances in diagnostic imaging and overstimations of disease prevalence and the benefits of therapy. N Engl J Med 1993;328:1237–1243.

6. Smith DS, Catalona WJ. The nature of prostate cancer detected through prostate specific antigen based screening. J Urol 1994;152:1732–1736.

7. Mettlin C, Murphy GP, Lee F, et al. Characteristics of prostate cancers detected in a multimodality early detection program. Cancer 1993;72:1701–1708.

8. Mueller CB. Breast cancer trials on trial: a case of conflicting ethical interests. Cancer 1995;75:2403–2406, 2410–2411. Editorial.

9. Lawrence W, Bear HD. Is there really an ethical conflict in clinical trials? Cancer 1995;75:2407–2409. Editorial.

10. Davis S, Wright PW, Schulman SF, et al. Participants in prospective, randomized clinical trials for resected non-small cell lung cancer have improved survival compared with nonparticipants in such trials. Cancer 1985;56:1710–1718.

11. Gleason DR. Histologic grade, clinical stage and patient age in prostate cancer. NCI Monogr 1988;7:15–18.

12. Prostate cancer incidence and mortality. J Natl Cancer Inst 1993; 85:1023.

13. Blute ML, Zincke H, Farrow GM. Long-term follow-up of young patients with stage A adenocarcinoma of the prostate. J Urol 1986; 136:840–843.

14. Stillwell TJ, Malek RS, Engen DE, Farrow GM. Incidental adenocarcinoma after open prostatic adenectomy. J Urol 1989;141:76–78.

15. Lowe BA, Barry JM. The predictive accuracy of staging transurethral resection of the prostate in the management of stage A cancer of the prostate: a comparative evaluation. J Urol 1990;143:1142–1145.

16. Greene DR, Egawa S, Neerhut G, et al. The distribution of residual cancer in radical prostatectomy specimens in stage A prostate cancer. J Urol 1991;145:324–329.

17. Whitmore WF, Warner JA, Thompson IM. Expectant management of localized prostatic cancer. Cancer 1991;67:1091–1096.

18. Lerner SP, Seale-Hawkins C, Carlton CR, Scardino PT. The risk of dying of prostate cancer in patients with clinically localized disease. J Urol 1991;146:1040–1045.

19. Adolfsson J, Steineck G, Whitmore WF. Recent results of management of palpable clinically localized prostate cancer. Cancer 1993;72:10–322.

20. Chodak GW, Thisted RA, Gerber GS, et al. Results of conservative management of clinically localized prostate cancer. N Engl J Med 1994;330:242–248.

21. Chodak GW. The role of conservative management in localized prostate cancer. Cancer 1994;74:2178–2181.

22. Loeb LA. Microsatellite instability: marker of a mutator phenotype in cancer. Cancer Res 1994;54:5059–5063.

23. Prehn RT. Cancers beget mutations versus mutations beget cancers. Cancer Res 1994;54:5296–5300.

24. Parsons R, Li GM, Longley M, et al. Mismatch repair deficiency in phenotypically normal human cells. Science 1995;268:738–740.

25. Markiewicz D, Hanks GE. Therapeutic options in the management of incidental carcinoma of the prostate. Int J Radiat Oncol Biol Phys 1991;20:153–167.

26. Johansson J-E, Adami HO, Andersson S-O, et al. High 10-year survival rate in patients with early, untreated prostatic cancer. JAMA 1992;267:2191–2196.

27. Fleming C, Wasson JH, Albertsen PC, et al. A decision analysis of alternative treatment strategies for clinically localized prostate cancer. JAMA 1993;269:2650–2658.

28. Kolata G. Advances in detection create dilemma on prostate cancer. New York Times, June 17, 1993.

29. Kolata G. Whether positive or negative result of prostate cancer test can create maze of questions. New York Times, June 23, 1993.

30. Mann CC. The prostate-cancer dilemma. Atlantic Monthly 1993;272:102–118.

31. Haapiainen R, Rannikko S, Makinen J, et al. T_0 carcinoma of the prostate: influence of tumor extent and histologic grade on prognosis of untreated patients. Eur Urol 1986;12:16–20.

32. Johansson J-E, Adami H-O, Andersson S-O, et al. Natural history of localised prostatic cancer: a population-based study in 223 untreated patients. Lancet 1989;1:799–803.

33. Zhang G, Wasserman NF, Sidi AM, et al. Long-term follow-up results after expectant management of stage A1 prostatic cancer. J Urol 1991;146:99–103.

34. Blackard CE, Mellinger GT, Gleason DF. Treatment of stage 1 carcinoma of the prostate: a preliminary report. J Urol 1971;106: 729–733.

35. Byar DP, VACUR Group. Survival of patients with incidentally found microscopic cancer of the prostate: results of a clinical trial of conservative treatment. J Urol 1972;108:908–912.

36. Catalona WJ. Treatment strategies for prostate cancer. JAMA 1993;270:1691–1692. Letter.

37. Aus G. Prostate cancer: mortality and morbidity after non-curative treatment with aspects on diagnosis and treatment. Scand J Urol Nephrol Suppl 1994;167:1–41.

38. McNeal JE, Bostwick DG, Kindrachuk PA, et al. Patterns of progression in prostate cancer. Lancet 1986;1:60–63.

39. Stamey TA, McNeal J, Freiha F, Redwine E. Morphometric and clinical studies on sixty-eight consecutive radical prostatectomies. J Urol 1988;139:1235–1241.

40. Epstein JI, Carmichael M, Partin AW, Walsh PC. Is tumor volume an independent predictor of progression following radical prostatectomy? A multivariate analysis of one hundred and eighty-five clinical stage B adenocarcinomas of the prostate with five years follow-up. J Urol 1993;149:1478–1481.

41. Epstein JI, Pizov G, Walsa PC. Correlation of pathologic findings with progression following radical retropubic prostatectomy. Cancer 1993;71:3582–3593.

42. Stamey TA, McNeal J. Adenocarcinoma of the prostate. In: Walsh P, Retick AB, Stamey TA, Vaughan ED Jr, eds. Campbell's urology. Philadelphia: WB Saunders 1992:1200–1201.

43. Stamey TA, Freiha F, McNeal J, et al. Localized prostate cancer: relationship of tumor volume to clinical significance for treatment of prostate cancer. Cancer 1993;71:933–938.

44. McNeal JE, Villers AA, Redwine EA, et al. Histologic differentiation cancer volume and pelvic lymph node metastasis in adenocarcinoma of the prostate. Cancer 1990;66:1225–1233.

45. Epstein J, Walsh P, Carmichael M, Brendler C. Pathologic and clinical findings to predict tumor extent in nonpalpable (stage T1c) prostate cancer. JAMA 1994;271:368–374.

46. Stamey TA. Prostate cancer: some basic clinical and morphometric observations in prostate cancer. Monogr Urol 1989;10:80.

47. Schmid HP, McNeal JE, Stamey TA. Observations on the doubling time of prostate cancer: the use of serial prostate specific antigen in patients

with untreated disease as a measure of increasing volume. Cancer 1993;71:2031–2040.

48. Egawa S, Go M, Kuwao S, et al. Long-term impact of conservative management of localized prostate cancer. Urology 1993;42:520–527.

49. Bostwick D. Gleason grading in prostatic needle biopsies. Am J Clin Pathol 1994;18:796–803.

50. Irwin MB, Trapasso JG. Identification of insignificant prostate cancers: analysis of pre-operative parameters. Urology 1994;44:862–868.

51. Terris M, Haney D, Johnstone I, et al. Prediction of prostate cancer volume using prostate specific antigen levels, transrectal ultrasound, and systemic sextant biopsies. Urology 1995;45:75–80.

52. Cupp M, Bostwick D, Myers R, Oesterling J. The volume of prostate cancer in the biopsy specimen cannot reliably predict the quantity of cancer in the radical prostatectomy specimen on an individual basis. J Urol 1995;153:1543–1548.

53. Humphrey PA, Baty J, Keetch D. Carcinoma extent in needle biopsies and matched avaudrants in radical prostatectomy specimens. Mod Pathol 1995;8:78A.

54. Stenman U, Oesterling J. Impact of tumor doubling time (DT) and age based reference values for PSA on prostate cancer (PCa) screening outcome. J Urol 1995;153:505A.

55. Stenman U, Knekt P, Arpo A. Serum PSA increases 6–10 years before diagnosis of prostate cancer. J Urol 1995;153:297A.

56. Outwater E, Peterson R, Siegelman E, et al. Prostate carcinoma: assessment of diagnostic criteria for capsular penetration on endorectal coil MR images. Radiology 1994;193:333–339.

57. Blute M, Ofner N, Zincke H, et al. Patterns of failure after radical retropubic prostatectomy for clinically localized adenocarcinoma of the prostate: influence of tumor DNA ploidy. J Urol 1989;142:1262–1265.

58. Greene D, Taylor S, Wheeler T, Scardino P. DNA ploidy by image analysis of individual foci of prostatic cancer: a preliminary report. Cancer Res 1991;51:4084–4089.

59. Hall M, Navone N, Trancoso P, et al. Frequency and characterization of p53 mutations in clinically localized prostate cancer. Urology 1995;45:470–475.

60. Meyers F, Chi SG, Fishman JR, et al. p53 mutations in benign prostatic hyperplasia. J Natl Cancer Inst 1993;85:1856–1858.

61. Gousse AE, Slawin K, Wheeler T, et al. A novel approach for detecting p53 mutations in heterogeneous prostate tissue samples using TA-cloning-PCR/SSCP. J Urol 1994;151:471A.

62. Catalona WJ, Smith DS, Ratliff TL, et al. Detection of organ-confined prostate cancer is increased through prostate-specific antigen-based screening. JAMA 1993;270:948–954.

63. Epstein JI, Walsh PC, Carmichael M, et al. Pathologic and clinical findings to predict tumor extent of non-palpable (stage T1c) prostate cancer. JAMA 1994;271:368–374.

64. Walsh PC. Prostate cancer kills: strategy to reduce deaths. Presented at the annual meeting of the American Urological Association, San Francisco, May 1994.

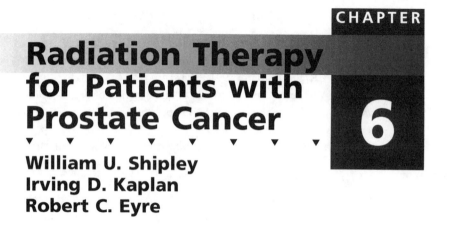

Radiation Therapy for Patients with Prostate Cancer

6

▼   ▼   ▼   ▼   ▼   ▼   ▼   ▼

William U. Shipley
Irving D. Kaplan
Robert C. Eyre

T wo radiation modalities are currently used in the treatment of early prostate cancer. The first and by far the most useful modality is external beam irradiation, using mainly high-energy photon or x-ray beams produced by linear accelerators. The second and less commonly used modality is interstitial isotopic radioactive seed implantation, using iodine-125 or palladium-103 radioactive sources.

■ TREATMENT TECHNIQUE

The modern era of external beam radiation was ushered in by Bagshaw and colleagues at Stanford University School of Medicine (1–3). Pelvic fields were used to treat the prostate and the pelvic lymph nodes and often the common iliac lymph nodes. This four-field volume receives 4,600 to 5,040 cGy using 180 to 200 cGy daily fractions, five sessions a week. The prostate tumor target volume is then raised 1,800 to 2,000 cGy, for a total dose to the primary tumor target volume of 6,400 to 7,040 cGy in seven to eight weeks. This technique has been well described by Bagshaw (2), and a composite isotope distribution curve of a representative treatment field is illustrated in Figure 6.1.

Hanks described the results of a large study of the manner in which external beam radiation was administered for prostate cancer in the United States in 1973 and 1974 and again in 1978 (4). This "Patterns of Care" study provides important data, as it represents a random sample of facilities throughout the United States, with the

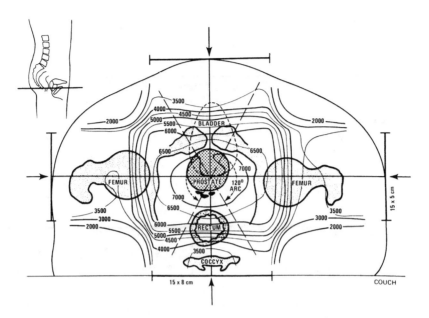

Fig. 6.1 *Composite isotope distribution of the radiation dose using external beam radiation therapy in a transverse cross section taken at the level of the prostate. (Reproduced with permission from Bagshaw MA, Cox RS, Ray GR. Status of radiation treatment of prostate cancer at Stanford University. NCI Monogr 1988;7:47.)*

results based on examination of more than 1,500 patient records. This audit data indicates that high-energy beams (those with energies equal to or greater than 6 MeV beams), complex field arrangement, and total radiation dose are all necessary for optimal results. Whether lymph node irradiation is beneficial, and for patients with which stages of tumor, has been a source of controversy for several years. The Radiation Therapy Oncology Group (RTOG) has analyzed data from a prospective trial that indicated that neither CT nor lymphangiogram was sufficiently accurate to rule out microscopic nodal disease in these men; the false-negative rate for these studies was likely to be at least 15% to 20% (5). Several retrospective studies have suggested that pelvic nodal radiation improves the disease-free survival (6,7), while two other studies, both of randomized comparisons, indicated no or only limited benefit (8,9). Pelvic nodal irradiation has been offered based on 1) patient tolerance, 2) the risk of lymph node involvement, and 3) institutional preference.

Over the past five years the development of sophisticated radiation-treatment-planning computers has allowed the three-dimensional visualization of the prostate and of the nearby normal structures (10–13). This localization makes it possible for the radiation oncologist to tailor radiation fields to the shape of the target tissue and thereby conform the high-dose volume only to structures judged to contain malignant cells and to exclude from the high-dose volume a significantly larger proportion of the anterior rectal wall and of the lower hemisphere of the bladder. Long-term results on treatment efficacy and normal tissue tolerance are not yet available, but the early results on radiation tolerance certainly suggest a reduction in acute urinary and rectal sequelae with 3-D conformal methods compared with conventional techniques. Based on studies of long-term outcome using conformal protons that demonstrate a reduction in late rectal bleeding when there is a reduction in the amount of anterior rectal wall raised to high dose (14), we can anticipate that the use of three-dimensional conformal techniques with linear accelerator beams will also be of long-term benefit to patients.

There is at present no consensus on the correct total dose to the prostate target volume by external beam radiation. However, based on analysis of both morbidity and treatment outcomes (see below), dosages in the range of 66.6 Gy to 70.2 Gy in 1.8-Gy daily fractions are now most commonly used in this country and are currently the dosages used in multi-institutional clinical trials by RTOG, the European Organization for the Research and Treatment of Cancer (EORTC), and the Southwestern Oncology Group (SWOG).

■ TREATMENT OUTCOME

Stages T1 and T2 Following External Beam Irradiation

Even though extensive data are available on outcome following irradiation for stage T1 and T2 prostate carcinoma, the results are difficult to compare because of heterogeneity of tumors within the reported study groups, differences in reported end points, and differences in methods of analysis. Such heterogeneity makes comparisons even of one radiation technique to another impossible. We are fortunate to have a Patterns of Care national database, which truly represents our national average of the results for patients treated with external beam radiation for T1 tumors. There is no excess mortality compared with the expected survival to 15 years based on both the Patterns of Care data and the RTOG data. These patients can be considered cured (15) (Fig. 6.2). The same data sets show that the patients with T2 tumors have a higher local recurrence rate (30% at 15 years) and show an excess of mortality of approximately 20% at 15 years post-therapy by analysis of hazard rates (15).

Serial follow-up PSA determination has revolutionized outcome reporting because of its objectivity and its sensitivity compared with clinical assessment. A rising PSA after therapy defines a biochemical relapse and is an accurate assessment of disease relapse. Many studies now with long-term "biochemical" follow-up of radiation-treated patients are being reported. These reports are summarized in

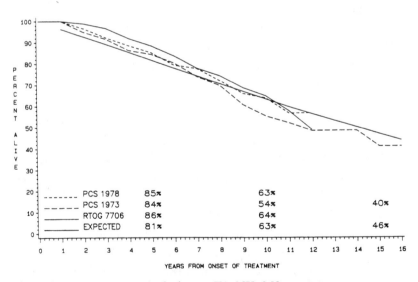

Fig. 6.2 *Long-term survival of stage T1, NX, M0 prostate cancer. Patients treated with radiation in the Pattern of Care studies (surveys 1973, 60 patients, and 1978, 115 patients) and in RTOG 77-06: 84 patients compared to expected survival. (Reproduced by permission from Hanks GE, Hanlon A, Schultheiss T, et al. Early prostate cancer: the national results of radiation treatment from the Patterns of Care and RTOG studies with prospects for improvement with conformal radiation and adjuvant androgen deprivation. J Urol 1994;152:1775–1780.)*

Table 6.1. Lee and Sause (16) report results of 91 node-negative patients treated with radiation, all with 15 years of follow-up. They reported 92% were free of local regrowth and that 62% were both clinically free of disease and free of PSA failure at 15 years. In the RTOG prospective trial of 104 patients with T1, T2, N0 tumors, 60% were clinically disease free at 10 years, and 39% are known to be surviving at 10 years with a PSA of less than 1.5 ng/mL (15). Schellhammer and colleagues (17) retrospectively analyzed 91 patients treated with radiation (69 by external beam and 22 by iodine-125 implantation); with biochemical control defined as a PSA level of less than 4 ng/mL, the disease-free status at 10 years was only 23% for external beam, but it was 90% for the implant treatment. These numbers were halved if an undetectable PSA was required to be disease-free. All the implant patients were surgically staged as N0, while for the external beam patients the nodal status was unknown. A higher percentage of implant patients were well differentiated (45% versus 26%). It is likely that the difference in patient inclusion or exclusion for one treatment or another based on tumor characteristics is the main factor explaining differences in outcome seen between these two groups. *This study underlines the great impact of selection by tumor characteristics in comparing outcome of any of the prostate cancer therapies.*

Bagshaw and colleagues present one of the most thorough and mature analyses of patient outcome with primary radiation for prostate cancer in the oncologic literature (18). It is unequaled for its sheer size (1,245 patients) and its 20 to 25 years of follow-up. Particularly impressive are the results for T1 to T2a patients of all grades. The 15-year overall survival rate is 48%, while the 15-year overall survival rate for those patients who were surgically staged as lymph node negative is 53%. This compares favorably with the 55% 15-year survival predicted for an age-matched population of controls without prostate cancer and with a match-pair comparison with surgery reported by Frehia from Stanford (19). No surgical or observation series has the high patient numbers or the long follow-up of the Bagshaw radiation series (18–20). Of all 377 patients with T1 to T2a tumors, only 28% died of prostate cancer in 20 years of follow-up. The Massachusetts General Hospital has recently reported (21) a series of

Table 6.1 Outcome with radiation therapy alone

Reference	Institution	Modality	No. Patients	Follow-up (yr)	Stage	Actuarial Disease-Free Survival
Hanks et al. (15)	RTOG	External beam	104	10	T1–2, N0	67% clinical[a]
Lee and Sause (16)	LDS	External beam	71	15	T1–2, N0	64% clinical[b]
		Implant	20			40% clinical[b]
Schellhammer et al. (17)	EVMS	External beam	69	10	T1b, NX	32% PSA <4
					T2a, NX	23%
		Implant	22	10	T1b, N0	76%
					T2a, N0	90%
Bagshaw et al. (18)	Stanford	External beam	377	15	T1–2a, NX	48% overall
		External beam	132	15	T1–2a, N0	53% overall
Frehia (19)	Stanford	External beam	53	10	T1–2c, N0	75% overall
Stamey et al. (20)	Stanford	External beam	98	6	44% T3–4 or N+	22%[c]
		Implant	15			
Colvert et al. (21)	Massachusetts General Hospital	External beam	196	8	T1–2a	46% PSA <4 / 33% PSA <1
Fowler et al. (22)	University of Mississippi	External beam	138	10	T1–2, NX	36% PSA rise

[a] 88% of these patients had a PSA <4.0ng/mL.
[b] Biochemical disease-free survival at 15 years is 62% for the combined group.
[c] Failure defined as a rising trend in PSA.
RTOG = Radiation Therapy Oncology Group
LDS = Latter Day Saints Hospital, Salt Lake City
EVMS = Eastern Virginia Medical School, Norfolk

196 patients with T1 to T2a N0/NX well to moderately differentiated tumors, with 8-year actuarial outcomes, overall survival (73%), cause-specific survival (85%), clinical local control (84%), and biochemical disease-free of rates of 46% (PSA less than 4.0 ng/mL) and 33% (PSA less than 1.0 ng/mL). Most recently the group from University of Mississippi reported results with external beam radiation therapy in 138 stage T1b to T2c NX patients. By actuarial calculations at 10 years, they report an overall survival rate of 35%, a cause-specific survival of 87%, and a PSA disease-free survival of 36% (22).

Morbidity of External Beam Irradiation

Although mild side effects during treatment, such as fatigue, urinary frequency and burning diarrhea, and occasional rectal bleeding may occur in up to one-half of patients while receiving irradiation, the complications described in Table 6.2 are those that persist beyond the first month after treatment is completed (23). All post-treatment sequelae of conventional external beam irradiation were mild to moderate (grades 2 and 3; there were no grade 4 or 5 complications). The only patient who became incontinent had had three preceding transurethral resections, two before and one following radiation therapy. The rate of rectal and bladder neck complications has been related to dose, field size, and the relative volume of organ irradiated (14,24). Therefore, with the newer techniques of 3-D conformal radiotherapy, the tumor volume can be more accurately localized, and the proportions of the adjacent organs that need to be raised to the dose given to the tumor is smaller. These efforts have resulted in lower proportions of patients with acute reactions with conventional and higher tumor doses (10,12,13). Thus, higher doses may be tolerated as well or better if smaller volumes of normal tissue need be treated with the higher doses given to the tumor.

Interstitial Radiotherapy for Stage T1 and T2 Tumors

The term *brachytherapy* literally means "close" therapy. With this technique, radioactive material is placed into tissues, which are treated as the material naturally decays. This is the oldest form of radiotherapy. In 1913 at the International Medical Congress, Section of Urology, Degrais presented a technique whereby a silver tube con-

Table 6.2 *Morbidity (grades 2 and 3) following external beam irradiation of T1–T2 prostate cancer (23)*

Patients evaluated	331
Median follow-up	6.1 years
Treatment mortality	0%
Grade 4 complications	0%
Incontinence	0.4%
Impotence	63% at 5 years
Diarrhea	
Incidence	3.6%
Persistence	0%
Rectal bleeding	
Incidence	5.4%
Persistence	0.6%
Hematuria	
Incidence	5.1%
Persistence	0.9%
Genitourinary strictures	
Incidence	5.4%
Persistence	1.2%

taining radium was introduced into the urethra. The pioneering American urologist H. H. Young brought this technique to the United States and refined it by placing radioactive sources into the prostate through the perineum. The results of the first 100 cases were reported in 1922 (25).

In the 1960s a method of implanting radioactive gold or iodine seeds was developed. With this approach, the radioactive material is permanently placed into the prostate via a retropubic approach, following a pelvic lymphadenectomy. In several reports the local control obtained by this method was compared with similarly staged patients treated with external beam radiation. Except for very early stage prostate cancer (T1b tumors), Koprowski, Kuban, and Morton reported inferior rates of local control using retropubic 125-iodine implantation (26–28). Morton and Wallner suggest that there was significant dose inhomogenety due to the nonuniformity of seed placement leading to underdosing of portions of the prostate gland (28,29).

Recently, transrectal ultrasonography (TRUS) has been used to visualize iodine-125 seed placement during transperineal implantation (30). A high dose of radiation is delivered to the prostate as the radioactive seeds decay. The early reported rates of serious late complications are much higher than with external beam therapy (29): a reported 8% rate of rectal ulceration with 3% of patients requiring colostomy. At two years after therapy, a 10% rate of grade 3 urinary complications (complications requiring surgery) was observed. Due to the rapid fall off of dose away from the implant, significantly less radiation is delivered to the periprostatic tissues. Consequently this technique is not indicated for men who are at risk for extracapsular extension of disease. Thus, only a small fraction of patients, perhaps 10%, should be considered for this approach—i.e., those with non-palpable tumors, without BPH, with relatively low pretherapy PSA levels, and with well-differentiated tumors.

Stages T3 and T4 Following Radiation Alone or Radiation Combined with Endocrine Therapy

When the cancer extends beyond the confines of the prostatic capsule, external beam radiation has been recommended as standard therapy, with the high-dose radiation volume encompassing the prostate, the seminal vesicles, and the periprostatic tissues. With reasonably low morbidity (24), the 10- and 15-year survival data from a large series of patients from Stanford (31), M. D. Anderson (32), Washington University (33), and the Patterns of Care studies (34) demonstrate that conventional external beam radiation therapy alone can result in the long-term survival of a small percentage of patients (Table 6.3). When progression is more precisely defined by a rising PSA level, there now is ample evidence that external beam radiation therapy alone for patients with T3 and T4 tumors can only infrequently prevent progression. Failure rates range from 85% at 5 years to up to 90% at 10 years (22,35–39). Similarly poor results using PSA criteria are seen with those few patients selected for treatment with surgical therapy alone (40,41).

Table 6.3 *The 10- and 15-year overall survival rates for patients with T3 and T4 prostate cancer treated with external beam radiotherapy alone*

Series	Tumor-Stage	Overall Survival	
		10 yr	*15 yr*
Stanford (31)	T3	35%	18%
	T4	15%	15%
M. D. Anderson (32)	T3	45%	31%
Washington University (33)	T3	42%	NS
Patterns of Care (34)	T3	33%	23%

NS = not stated.

These results have encouraged approaches that increase radiation dose without increasing the radiation complication rates to the bladder and rectum, using conformal radiotherapy techniques and by the addition of combined androgen deprivation. A recent single institutional randomized trial evaluating the effect of radiation dose escalation with radiation alone, comparing the standard dose of 67.2 Gy with a dose of 75.6 CGE (cobalt-Gy equivalent) using a conformal proton boost, resulted in no significant improvement in overall or relapse-free survival (37). However, there appeared to be benefit in local control at eight years in the high-dose versus conventional-dose arm (77% versus 60%, $p = 0.089$). Several centers are now exploring dose escalations using these techniques up to and beyond 80 Gy but as yet have not submitted such an approach to a comparative randomized trial (42–49). Neutron beam therapy deposits significantly more energy per unit of transversed tissue and thus has more severe biologic consequences of dose and the radiation damage is less dependent on tissue oxygenation. The Neutron Therapy Collaborative Working Group has recently reported its second randomized trial in patients with T3 and T4 tumors, comparing high-energy photons to neutrons (45). The group reports improvement in preventing local regrowth of the tumor (87% versus 68%). However, there was no improvement in overall or cause-specific survival, and a significantly higher incidence of major complications in the neutron group was reported.

Castration was shown in the 1940s to cause regression of prostatic tissue of prostatic cancer. Androgen ablation is associated with an inhibition of cell proliferation and with activation of programmed cell death by apoptosis. Since the rate of tumor cure with radiation therapy increases with a reduction in tumor size, the reduction in tumor bulk induced by androgen deprivation likely will increase the probability of eradication of a subsequently irradiated tumor. Recently the RTOG has evaluated by randomized trials the combining of radiation therapy with androgen deprivation. Patients with bulky primary tumors were treated by radiation alone or radiation in combination with four months of androgen suppression. The androgen suppression therapy was two months of goserelin acetate (Zoladex) and flutamide (Eulexin) before and two months during radiation therapy. With a median potential follow-up of four and a half years, a sig-nificant improvement in the progression-free survival rate was seen at five years for combined modality therapy versus radiation alone (36% versus 15%, $p < 0.001$). The advantages of short-term androgen deprivation with radiation therapy have not as yet translated into an overall survival advantage, although this is expected with longer observation (38).

The RTOG has also recently reported results of another randomized trial studying adjuvant androgen suppression following radiation in patients with very poor risk but apparently locally, or at least regionally, confined prostate cancer. This trial accrued 950 patients and should be able to see a 10% or greater survival benefit, if it is present. With a median follow-up of only three years, this study is showing a significant benefit in preventing local regrowth of the tumor and, as expected, a significant benefit in progression-free survival using a PSA end point of 1.5 ng/mL or greater as evidence of progression (46,47). A summary of these two trials is shown in Table 6.4.

Based on the results of the recently reported randomized trials (37,38,45,46) and many other single institutional series, the practice of monotherapy for patients with T3 prostatic cancer by radical prostatectomy (40,41), radiation therapy (31–34,39), or only androgen ablation alone, with the intent of curing the patient, should be abandoned. Nevertheless, with combined modality therapy, patients pre-

Table 6.4 *Results to date of two recently reported Radiation Therapy Orcology Group (RTOG) comparative randomized trials of radiation alone versus combined modality treatment with radiation and endocrine therapy in patients with advanced prostate cancer*

Randomized Trial	Stage	No. Randomized Patients	Local Treatment	No Evidence of Local Regrowth[a]	With PSA	Survival Overall
RTOG 8610	cT3–T4 (≥25 cm^2)	456	XRT	32%	15%	71%
			MAB[b] + XRT	13%	36%	71%
				($p < 0.001$)	($p < 0.001$)	($p = 0.7$)
RTOG 85-31	cT3 (<25 cm^2);	950	XRT	32%	17%	71%
	cT1–T3, pN+;		XRT + HT[c]	17%	49%	76%
	pT3			($p < 0.001$)	($p < 0.001$)	($p = 0.39$)

[a] No evidence of disease using serial PSA in follow-up.

[b] Maximal androgen blockage for four months, two before and two during XRT; goserelin (Zoladex) 3.6 mg subcutaneously every four weeks and flutamide (Eulexin) 250 mg by mouth three times a day.

[c] Adjuvant hormone therapy, goserelin (Zoladex) 3.6 mg subcutaneously every four weeks.

XRT = external beam radiation therapy, conventional fractionation and doses; MAB = maximal androgen blockage; HT = hormone therapy.

PT3 = pathologic stage following radical prostatectomy

PN+ = pathologic stage following pelvic lymph node sampling.

senting with locally advanced disease may well have a realistic chance of cure if they are willing to accept the increased risks of side effects and symptoms from multimodality therapy and from higher than conventional doses of radiation.

Salvage Prostatectomy Following Radiation Therapy

Local persistence of tumor following radiation for localized prostatic cancer presents a clinically important and not uncommon dilemma. Salvage surgical procedures may still offer the potential cure to a *carefully selected* group of patients. For patients with stage T1 and T2 tumors, the clinically observed 10- and 15-year freedom from local tumor regrowth rates are excellent. However, subclinical local tumor persistence is likely in 20% to 30% of all irradiated patients. Prostate rebiopsies, especially in the setting of a rising postirradiation PSA, are now able to diagnose subclinical persistence of tumor when it is likely to be confined to the organ and amenable to surgical correction (surgical removal). The most recent results indicate success in salvaging a patient with persistent tumor when it is by pathologic staging still confined to the organ. Salvage prostatectomy is best carried out in men with original clinical stage T1 or T2 tumors that at the time of detection are still clinically confined to the gland and at a time when the patient's PSA is less than 10 ng/mL (48,49). The Baylor Group (48) reported that when salvage prostatectomy was done in patients with a PSA of less than 10 ng/mL or more than 10 ng/mL the non-progression rates are significantly ($p < .05$) better, 50% and 29%, respectively. However, the potential complication rates reported in salvage radical prostatectomy, even in contemporary series from experienced institutions (48–50), are higher than those done on unirradiated patients: i.e., rectal injury (0% to 20%), urinary incontinence (10% to 58%), lower extremity edema (up to 10%), and impotency (almost universal). The disease-free survival following salvage surgical therapy in contemporary series (48–52) ranges from 55% to 95% at 5 years and from 33% to 76% at 10 years. Some of the patients in these series also had androgen deprivation therapy following salvage surgery. The 5- and 10-year cancer-specific survival was reported from the Mayo Clinic as 92% and 76%, respectively (49). Given the above information, patients should have PSA levels assessed routinely every three to six months after radiation therapy. The PSA should normalize to a nadir within the normal range or below within one to two years following radiation (53,54). Once the PSA begins to rise following normalization (to more than 1.0 ng/mL above the nadir value), younger patients should be evaluated for salvage surgery. However, these patients should also be highly motivated for cure and have a 10-year life expectancy and a positive prostate rebiopsy. Optimally these patients should originally have been clinical stage T1 or T2, with moderately or well-differentiated tumors with a PSA still within the normal range or certainly less than 10 ng/mL. It is this subgroup for whom early radical prostatectomy has the greatest likelihood of producing excellent local control, long-term survival, and possibly cure.

Radiation Therapy for Palliation of Symptoms from Metastatic Disease

Initial therapy for metastatic prostate cancer is usually androgen deprivation. However, although effective, its response is usually limited to two to five years, and then the disease progresses. Prostate cancer has a remarkable predilection to metastasize to bone. The symptomatic impact on a patient of progressive bone metastases should not be underestimated. It is projected that more than 40,000 men will die of metastatic prostate cancer in the United States in 1996, and the vast majority will have extensive bone disease. Bone pain is the most common pain syndrome observed in metastatic disease. Pathologic fracture of bone, especially weight-bearing bone, can occur with cortical erosion (55), adding to the morbidity of bone metastases. Metastatic deposits in the vertebral column can extrude, leading to spinal cord compression with devastating neurologic sequelae.

Pain relief following treatment can be difficult to evaluate and to quantitate. External beam radiotherapy is successful in reducing pain in approximately 80% of the sites treated (56,57). Different dose fractionation schemes have been evaluated. Blitzer reevaluated the results of the RTOG trial, testing various fractionation schedules, and reported that higher dose regimens (i.e., more lower dose fractions administered over a longer treatment time) provided a more durable response (58). However, the additional treatment time required to deliver therapy (e.g., one week versus two weeks versus four weeks of daily therapy) must be weighed against the effort involved in protracted schedules for patients with limited life expectancy.

Since patients with metastatic disease often develop diffuse sites of pain, large-field regional radiotherapy has been evaluated. With this technique entire regions are sequentially treated, with the goal of irradiating nearly the entire skeleton. In an RTOG trial, the upper hemibody was irradiated and subsequently the lower body was treated (59). In this study, 73% of patients received some relief, with 20% reporting complete relief from pain. Toxicity reactions such as myelosuppression, diarrhea, and pneumonitis were observed, especially in patients who had received prior chemotherapy. Kaplan and colleagues retrospectively observed a reduction in metastases in sites of prior incidental radiation exposure (60). This observation suggests that modest doses to the spine earlier in a patient's course when bone metastases are not too extensive may be of benefit.

Recently bone-seeking radiopharmaceuticals have been reintroduced into clinical practice. Bone-seeking radiopharmaceuticals are well suited for metastatic prostate cancer. These compounds attempt to exploit the high rate of blastic bone disease observed with prostate cancer. 32-Phosphorous was shown to have a clinical response in treating metastatic prostate cancer. However, hematologic toxicity limited its usefulness. Other radiopharmaceuticals, including 186-rhenium (Rh), 153-Semenarium (Sm), and 89-strontium (Sr), have been tested. 89-Sr has been approved for use for metastatic cancer in the United States. Strontium has chemical characteristics similar to calcium and will preferentially deposit at sites of active bone remodeling, such as areas of blastic metastatic disease.

Several major trials have been conducted to test the efficacy of 89-Sr. In a British and Canadian multicenter trial, response to therapy was assessed at 12 weeks after administration of 89-Sr. Response was determined by patient report, assessment of patient mobility, and narcotic requirement (61). Fifty-five percent of the 83 patients reported a substantial response to treatment; better responses were observed in patients with less extensive disease determined by bone scan intensity. In another multicenter trial with a crossover design (radioactive strontium versus natural strontium), 26 patients were treated with some short-term pain palliation (62). The Trans Canada 89-Sr Study demonstrated a significantly lower analgesic requirement, and a lower rate of additional external beam irradiation treatments than the control group. Quality of life and patient activity were superior in the patients receiving 89-Sr (63).

In summary, the treatment of symptomatic bone metastases is critical for maintaining the quality of life in patients with metastatic prostate cancer. The importance of palliative care in maintaining the patient at the highest functional status should not be underestimated. In addition to analgesic medication or other therapies, radiotherapeutic intervention usually is of great palliative benefit.

Editorial Comment

Radiation therapy for prostate cancer is an effective treatment. A great deal of experience has been acquired using external beam radiation. More recently brachytherapy, or radioactive seed implantation, has become popular. In general, patients who are treated with radiation therapy, particularly external beam radiation, tend to be older, to have greater comorbidity, and to have more advanced disease. In the absence of randomized trials, it is therefore difficult to make head-to-head comparisons of this treatment versus other forms of treatment. Radiation is chosen by or for such patients because of its relatively favorable treatment-related side effect profile. Radiation therapy will be adequate treatment for many patients. Radioactive implants provide an attractive alternative for patients with very minimal tumors and with small prostate glands; however, long-term efficacy is still unknown. The use of hormonal therapy in conjunction with radiation is being tested, although its long-term benefits are uncertain. In the treatment of symptomatic bone metastases radiation in addition to analgestic medication is usually of great palliative benefit.

■ **REFERENCES**

1. Bagshaw MA, Kaplan HS, Sagerman RH. Linear accelerator supervoltage radiotherapy VII: carcinoma of the prostate. Radiology 1965;85:121.

2. Bagshaw MA, Cox RS, Ray GR. Status of radiation treatment of prostate cancer at Stanford University. NCI Monogr. 1988;7:47.

3. Bagshaw MA. Carcinoma of the prostate. In: Levitt SH, ed. Technologic basis of radiotherapy: practical clinical applications. 2nd ed. Philadelphia: Lea & Febiger, 1992:300–322.

4. Hanks GE. External-beam radiation therapy for clinically localized prostate cancer: Patterns of Care studies in the United States. NCI Monogr. 1988;7:75.

5. Hanks GE, Krall JM, Pilepich MV, et al. Comparison of pathologic and clinical evaluation of lymph nodes in prostate cancer: implications of RTOG data for patient management and trial design and stratification. Int J Radiat Oncol Biol Phys 1992;23:293–298.

6. McGowan DG. The value of extended field radiation therapy in carcinoma of the prostate. Int J Radiat Oncol Biol Phys 1981;7:1333–1339.

7. Bagshaw MA. Potential for radiotherapy alone in prostatic cancer. Cancer 1985;55:2079–2085.

8. Spaas PG, Bagshaw MA, Cox RS. The value of extended field irradiation in surgically staged carcinoma of the prostate. Int J Radiat Oncol Biol Phys 1988;15(suppl 1):133–134.

9. Asbell SO, Krall JM, Pilepich MV, et al. Elective pelvic irradiation in stage A2, B carcinoma of the prostate: analysis of RTOG 77-06. Int J Radiat Oncol Biol Phys 1988;15:1307–1316.

10. Sofen EM, Hanks GE, Hwang CC, Chu JCH. Conformal static field therapy for low volume, low grade prostate cancer with rigid mobilization. Int J Radiat Oncol Biol Phys 1991;20:141–146.

11. Biggs BJ, Shipley WU. A beam width improving device for a 25 MV x-ray beam. Int J Radiat Oncol Biol Phys 1986;12:131–135.

12. Ten Haken RK, Perez-Tamayo C, Tesser JR, et al. Boost treatment of the prostate using shaped, fixed fields. Int J Radiat Oncol Biol Phys 1989;16:193–200.

13. Vijayakumar S, Awan A, Karrison T, et al. Acute toxicity during external beam radiotherapy for localized prostatic cancer: comparison of different techniques. Int J Rad Oncol Biol Phys 1993;25:359.

14. Benk VA, Adams JA, Shipley WU, et al. Late rectal bleeding following combined x-ray and proton high dose irradiation for patients with stages T_3-T_4 prostate carcinoma. Int J Radiat Oncol Biol Phys 1993; 26:551–557.

15. Hanks GE, Hanlon A, Schultheiss T, et al. Early prostate cancer: the national results of radiation treatment from the Patterns of Care and RTOG studies with prospects for improvement with conformal radiation and adjuvant androgen deprivation. J Urol 1994;152:1775–1780.

16. Lee RJ, Sause WT. Surgically staged patients with prostate carcinoma treated with definitive radiation therapy: 15-year results. Urology 1994;43:640–644.

17. Schellhammer PF, El-Mahdi AM, Wright GL, et al. Prostate-specific antigen to determine progression-free survival after radiation therapy for localized carcinoma of the prostate. Urology 1993;42:13.

18. Bagshaw MA, Cox RS, Hancock SL. Control of prostate cancer with radiotherapy: long-term. J Urol 1994;152:1781–1785.

19. Frehia FS. A comparative study of external beam irradiation teletherapy and radical retropubic prostatectomy in men with clinically localized prostate cancer and pathologically negative lymph nodes: 10-year follow-up. In: Khoury S, Murphy GP, Chatelaine C, Denis L, eds. Proceedings of the Fourth International Symposium on Recent Advances in Urologic Cancer. Paris: Medical Edition Publishers, 1995:221–224.

20. Stamey TA, Ferrari MK, Schmid HP. The value of serial prostate specific antigen determinations 5 years after radiotherapy: steeply increasing values characterize 80% of patients. J Urol 1993;150:1856–1859.

21. Colvett KT, Zietman AL, Shipley WU. Radiation therapy for patients with T1 and T2a (B1) prostate cancer: selection yields high success rates maintained more than 10 years after treatment. In: Khoury S, Murphy GP, Chatelaine C, Denis L, eds. Proceedings of the Fourth International Symposium on Recent Advances in Urologic Cancer. Paris, Medical Edition Publishers, 1995:214–220.

22. Fowler JE Jr, Braswell NT, Pandey P, Seaver L. Experience with radical prostatectomy and radiation therapy for localized prostatic cancer at a Veterans Affairs Medical Center. J Urol 1995;153:1026–1031.

23. Shipley WU, Zietman AL, Hanks GE, et al. Treatment-related sequelae following external beam radiation therapy for prostate cancer: a review with update in patients with T1–2 tumors. J Urol 1994;152:1799–1805.

24. Lawton CA, Won M, Pilepich MV, et al. Long-term treatment sequelae following irradiation for adenocarcinoma of the prostate: analysis of RTOG studies 7506 and 7706. Int J Radiat Oncol Biol Phys 1991;21:935–940.

25. Young HH. Technique of radium treatment of cancer of the prostate and seminal vesicles. Surg Gynecol Obstet 1922;34:93–98.

26. Koprowski CD, Berkenstock KG, Borofski AM, et al. External beam irradiation versus 125-iodine implant in definitive treatment of prostate cancer. Int J Radiat Oncol Biol Phys 1991;21:955–960.

27. Kuban DA, Anas EM, Schellhammer PF. I-125 interstitial implantation for prostate cancer: what have we learned 10 years later? Cancer 1989;63:2415–2420.

28. Morton JD, Peschel RE. Iodine-125 implants versus external beam therapy for stage A2, B and C prostate cancer. Int J Radiat Oncol Biol Phys 1988;14:1153–1157.

29. Wallner K, Roy J, Zelefsky M, et al. Short-term freedom from disease progression after I-125 prostate implantation. Int J Radiat Oncol Biol Phys 1988;14:1153–1157.

30. Blasko JC, Grimm PD, Ragde H. Brachytherapy and organ preservation in the mangement of carcinoma of the prostate. Semin Radiat Oncol 1993;3:240–249.

31. Bagshaw MA, Kaplan ID, Cox RC. Radiation therapy for localized disease. Cancer 1993;71:939–952.

32. Zagars GK, von Escenbach AC, Ayala AG. Prognostic factors in prostate cancer: analysis of 874 patients treated with radiation therapy. Cancer 1993;72:1709–1725.

33. Perez CA, Lee HK, Georgiou A, et al. Technical and tumor-related factors affecting outcome of definitive irradiation for localized carcinoma of the prostate. Int J Radiat Oncol Biol Phys 1993;26:581–591.

34. Holmes GE, Krall JM, Hanton AL, et al. Patterns of care and RTOG studies in prostate cancer: Long-term survival, hazard rate observations and possibilities of cure. Int J Radiat Oncol Biol Phys 1993;28:39–45.

35. Dugan TC, Shipley WU, Young RH, et al. Biopsy after external beam radiation therapy for adenocarcinoma of the prostate: correlation with original histological grade and current prostate specific antigen levels. J Urol 1991;146:1313.

36. Kaplan ID, Bagshaw MA. Serum prostate-specific antigen after post-prostatectomy radiotherapy. Urology 1992;39:401–406.

37. Shipley WU, Verhey LJ, Munzenrider JE, et al. Advanced prostate cancer: the results of a randomized comparative trial of high dose irradiation boosting with conformal protons compared with conventional dose irradiation using photons alone. Int J Radiat Oncol Biol Phys 1995;32:3–12.

38. Pilepich MV, Krall JM, Al-Sarraf M, et al. Androgen suppression with radiation therapy compared with radiation therapy alone for locally advanced prostatic carcinoma: a randomized comparative trial of the Radiation Therapy Oncology Group. Urology 1995;45:616–623.

39. Kuban DA, El-Mahdi AM, Schellhammer PF. Prostate-specific antigen for pre-treatment prediction and post-treatment evaluation of outcome after definitive irradiation for prostate cancer. Int J Radiat Oncol Biol Phys 1995;32:307–316.

40. Morgan WR, Bergstralh EJ, Zincke H. Long-term evaluation of radical prostatectomy as treatment for clinical stage C (T3) prostate cancer. Urology 1993;41:113–120.

41. Van den Ouden D, Davidson PJT, Hop W, Schroeder FH. Radical prostatectomy as a monotherapy for locally advanced (stage T3) prostate cancer. J Urol 1994;151:646–651.

42. Sandler HM, Perez-Tamayo C, Ten Haken RK, Lichter AS. Dose escalation for stage C (T3) prostate cancer: minimal rectal toxicity observed using conformal therapy. Radiother Oncol 1992;23:53–54.

43. Leibel SA, Heimann R, Kuthcher GJ, et al. Three-dimensional conformal radiation therapy in locally advanced carcinoma of the prostate: preliminary results of a phase I dose escalation study. Int J Radiat Oncol Biol Phys 1993;28:55–65.

44. Schultheiss TE, Hanks GE, Hunt MA, et al. Incidence of and factors related to late complications in conformal and conventional radiation treatment of cancer of the prostate. Int J Radiat Oncol Biol Phys 1995;32:643–649.

45. Russell KJ, Caplan RJ, Laramore GE, et al. Photon versus fast neutron external beam radiotherapy in the treatment of locally advanced prostate cancer: results of a randomized prospective trial. Int J Radiat Oncol Biol Phys 1993;28:47–54.

46. Pilepich MV, Caplan R, Byhardt RW, et al. A phase III trial of androgen suppression using goserelin (Zoladex) in unfavorable prognosis of carcinoma of the prostate treated with definitive radiotherapy (report of RTOG protocol 85-31). Proc Am Soc Clin Oncol 1995;14:239. Abstract.

47. Pilepich MV. Combined radiation therapy and endocrine therapy in locally advanced prostate cancer. In: Vogelzang NJ, Scardino PT, Shipley WU, Coffey DS, eds. Comprehensive Textbook of Genitourinary Oncology. Baltimore: Williams & Wilkins, 1996:798–802.

48. Rogers E, Ohori, Kassabian VS, et al. Salvage radical prostatectomy: outcome measured by serum PSA levels. J Urol 1995;153:104–110.

49. Lerner SE, Blute ML, Zincke H. Critical evaluation of salvage surgery for radio-recurrent/resistant prostate cancer. J Urol 1995;154:1103–1109.

50. Pontes JE. Role of surgery in managing recurrence following external-beam radiation therapy. Urol Clin North Am 1994;21:701–706.

51. Moul JW, Paulson DF. The role of radical surgery in the management of radiation recurrent and large volume prostate cancer. Cancer 1991; 68:1265.

52. Ahlering TE, Lieskovsky G, Skinner DG. Salvage surgery plus androgen deprivation for radio resistant prostatic adenocarcinoma. J Urol 1992;147:900.

53. Kaplan ID, Cox RS, Bagshaw MA. Prostate specific antigen after external beam radiotherapy for prostatic cancer: follow-up. J Urol 1993; 149:519–522.

54. Willett CG, Zietman AL, Shipley WU, Coen JJ. The effect of pelvic irradiation therapy on the production of prostatic specific antigen. J Urol 1994;151:1579–1581.

55. Fidler M. Incidence of fracture through metastases in long bones. Acta Orthop Scand 1973;52:282–288.

56. Tong D, Gillick L, Hendrickson FR. The palliation of symptomatic osseous metastases: final results of the study by the Radiation Therapy Oncology Group. Cancer 1982;50:893–899.

57. Cole DJ. A randomized trial of a single treatment versus conventional fractionation in the palliative radiotherapy of painful bone metastases. J Clin Oncol 1989;1:59–62.

58. Blitzer PH. Reanalysis of the RTOG study of the palliation of symptomatic osseous metastasis. Cancer 1985;55:1468–1472.

59. Salazar OM, Rubin P, Hendrickson FR, et al. Single-dose half-body irradiation for palliation of multiple bone metastases from solid tumor. Cancer 1986;58:29–37.

60. Kaplan ID, Valdagni R, Cox RS, Bagshaw MA. Reduction of spinal metastases after preemptive irradiation in prostatic cancer. Int J Radiat Oncol Biol Phys 1990;18:1019–1025.

61. Laing AH, Ackery DM, Bayly RJ, et al. Stronium-89 chloride for pain palliation in prostatic skeletal malignancy. Br J Radiol 1991;64:816–822.

62. Lewington JH, McEwan AJ, Ackery DM, et al. A prospective randomized double-blind crossover study to examine the efficacy of stronium-89 in pain palliation in patients. Eur J Cancer 1991;27:954–958.

63. Porter AT, McEwan AJB, Powe JE, et al. Results of a randomized phase-III trial to evaluate the efficacy of strontium-89 adjuvant to local field external beam irradiation in the management of endocrine resistant metastatic prostate cancer. Int J Radiat Oncol Biol Phys 1993;25:805–813.

Radical Prostatectomy in the Treatment of Prostate Cancer

7

▼ ▼ ▼ ▼ ▼ ▼ ▼ ▼

Kevin R. Loughlin
Robert C. Eyre
Anthony L. Zietman

H UGH HAMPTON YOUNG first performed his radical perineal prostatectomy technique on a patient on April 7, 1904, with William H. Halsted assisting him (1). For the next 40 years radical perineal prostatectomy was the surgical treatment of choice for localized prostate cancer. Young reported in 1945 a nearly 50% cure rate in cases of localized prostate cancer followed from 5 to 27 years (1). Victor Marshall went on to say that "the only known cure for prostatic carcinoma is total excision" (2). However, in the mid-1940s Millin introduced the retropubic approach for the removal of the prostate (3). In the following 10 years Memmelar (4), Lattimer (5), and Chute (6) followed Millin's lead and popularized the retropubic approach as the means to perform a radical prostatectomy.

The surgical treatment of prostate cancer remained fairly static for almost another 40 years, until the publication of Walsh's technique for nerve-sparing retropubic prostatectomy (7). The publication of Walsh's technique resulted in a resurgence of interest in applying radical surgery for cure in the treatment of localized prostate cancer. Over the following decade, radical prostatectomy emerged as the preferred treatment for organ-confined prostate cancer. Goluboff and Olsson estimated that approximately 52,000 radical prostatectomies were performed in 1992 (8). Clearly, much has changed regarding the treatment of prostate cancer since Young's early report. In this chapter we will give an overview

119
▼

of the application of radical prostatectomy in the treatment of prostate cancer.

■ PATIENT SELECTION

The ideal patient for a radical prostatectomy is one who has organ-confined disease, is healthy enough to tolerate surgery, and is young enough to benefit from cure. In a practical sense, however, it is not always easy to rigidly apply these criteria to an individual patient. Although the treatment of each patient must be individualized, certain guidelines are useful.

Age

The patient's chronologic age alone cannot be used as the sole criterion to determine whether he is a surgical candidate; however, it must be factored in to the decision. McLaughlin has advised that age 72 is a reasonable cutoff point beyond which men should not be considered candidates for radical prostatectomy (9). Middleton and Larsen have advocated taking the patient's likely life expectancy into account when deciding whether radical prostatectomy is a good therapeutic option (10). They recommend utilizing life expectancy as estimated in a table from the National Center for Health Statistics (Table 7.1).

Table 7.1 *Average life expectancy among white American men, 1986 (National Center for Health Statistics)*

Age (yr)	Average Years Remaining
65	14.8
70	11.7
75	9.1
80	6.9

SOURCE: Reproduced by permission from Middleton RG, Larsen RG. Selection of patients with stage B prostate cancer for radical prostatectomy. Urol Clin North Am 1990;17:779–785.

Stage

The topic of preoperative staging is discussed in Chapter 3 of this book. Physical exam, tumor markers, ultrasound, CT scan, MRI, and bone scan may all contribute to more accurate preoperative staging. Regardless of which modalities are used for staging, there is a growing consensus among physicians who treat prostate cancer that radical surgery is best reserved for patients with organ-confined disease (stage A, B or T1, T2). Although surgical cures can be achieved for stage C (T3) disease (11–15) and stage D1 (N1–N2) disease (16–21), the best results have consistently been achieved in patients with disease confined to the prostate. Table 7.2 is adapted from Austenfeld and Davis (16), and it demonstrates that the mean time to progression in several large series of stage D1 (N1–N2) patients treated with radical prostatectomy alone ranged from 18.3 to 58.8 months and that disease-free survival ranged from 18.5 to 75 months.

Tumor Markers

Tumor markers are discussed more fully in Chapters 3 and 5. However, it is important to reiterate that preoperative prostate-specific

Table 7.2 *Time to progression and survival rates in stage D1 prostatic cancer*

Source*	No. Patients	Mean Age (yr)	Mean Time to Progression (mo)	Months of Follow-up (range)	Disease-Free Survival (%) 5 yr	Disease-Free Survival (%) 5–10 yr
Kramer et al. 1981 (17)	11	62.0	18.3	—	—	—
Utz 1984 (18)	52	63.0	—	(6–180)	18.5	—
Myers et al. 1988 (19)	38	62.1	45.6	95.0 (76–229)	21.0	—
Zincke 1989 (20)	104	63.7	55.0	56.4 (1–252)	48.0	38
Catalona et al. 1988 (21)	12	62.0	58.8	72.0 (48–120)	75.0	36

* Patients treated with surgery alone.

SOURCE: Modified from Austenfeld MS, Davis BE. New concepts in the treatment of stage D-1 adenocarcinoma of the prostate. Urol Clin North Am 1990;17:867–884.

antigen (PSA) is useful in selecting patients who are most likely to benefit from surgery.

Oesterling and colleagues (22) evaluated preoperative prostate-specific antigen as a predictor of pathologic stage found at the time of radical prostatectomy in 178 consecutive patients. Although PSA correlated directly with capsular penetration ($p < 0.002$), seminal vesicle involvement ($p < 0.02$), and lymph node involvement ($p < 0.05$), the diagnostic accuracy of an elevated PSA on an individual basis was only 55% for capsular penetration and 50% for seminal vesicle involvement. Their data are reproduced in Figure 7.1. What is most striking is the degree of overlap between organ- and nonorgan-confined disease in the lower PSA ranges.

A similar study was performed by Hudson and associates (23). They analyzed PSA in 231 men with prostate cancer. Of the 103 men with stage A or B (T1, T2) organ-confined disease, 36% had PSA levels greater than 10. Although there was a trend of increasing PSA levels with higher clinical stage, there again was considerable overlap. Their data appear in Figure 7.2.

A further study by Lange (24) generated a PSA table that could be used to predict the likelihood of tumor extension to the seminal vesicles or lymph nodes. His data are reproduced in Table 7.3.

Given these limitations of PSA in accurately predicting pathologic stage, Partin and colleagues (25) examined the utility of combining clinical stage, Gleason score, and PSA in predicting pathologic stage in 703 patients with clinically localized prostate cancer. They found that the three parameters taken together were better than any individual parameter alone in predicting pathologic stage. The probability plots and nomograms generated from their study appear in Figures 7.3 and 7.4. They reported that 75% of the men with a serum PSA value less than 4.0 ng/mL had organ-confined disease. In men with PSA between 4.0 and 10.0 ng/mL, only 53% had organ-confined disease. Furthermore, only 2 of 28 men with PSA levels greater than 30 ng/mL had organ-confined disease.

Prostate acid phosphatase (PAP) has fallen into relative disuse with the advent of PSA. This has been mainly due to the fact that PAP cross-reacts with serum acid phosphatase from other tissues (26). In addition, both radioimmunoassay and enzymatic PAP assays are not

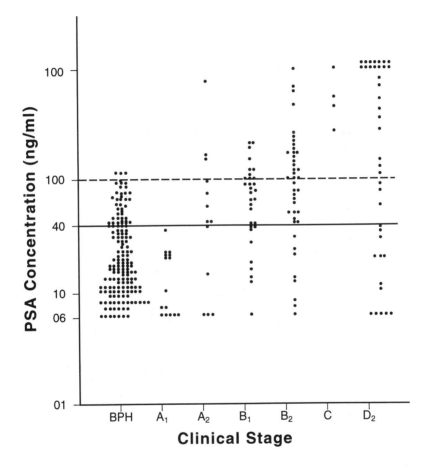

Fig. 7.1 *Plot of preoperative PSA values with respect to pathology of the prostate. BPH = benign prostatic hyperplasia, CP = capsular penetration, SV = seminal vesicle involvement, LN = lymph node involvement.*

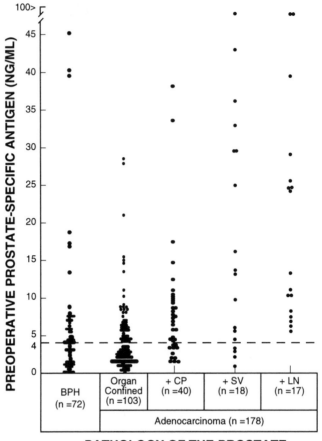

Fig. 7.2 *Preoperative PSA values in patients with benign prostatic hyperplasia (BPH) and prostate cancer stages A to D.*

sensitive or specific in identifying organ-confined disease (27). Prostatic acid phosphatase determinations are no longer routinely performed by most urologists in the United States.

Radiographic Studies

The role of radiographic studies in selecting patients who are good surgical candidates is fully discussed in Chapter 3 and will not be reiterated here. It is important to realize that the role of the preoper-

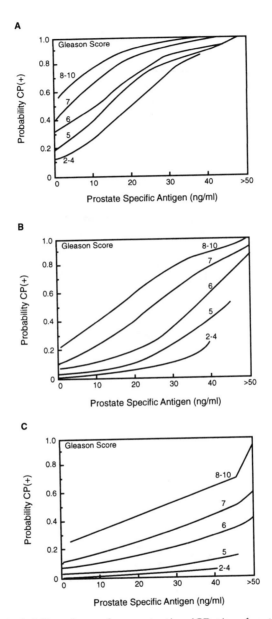

Fig. 7.3 *A) Probability of capsular penetration (CP+) as function of serum PSA and preoperative Gleason score. B) Probability of seminal vesicle involvement (SV+) as function of serum PSA and preoperative Gleason score. C) Probability of lymph nodel involvement (LN+) as function of serum PSA and preoperative Gleason score.*

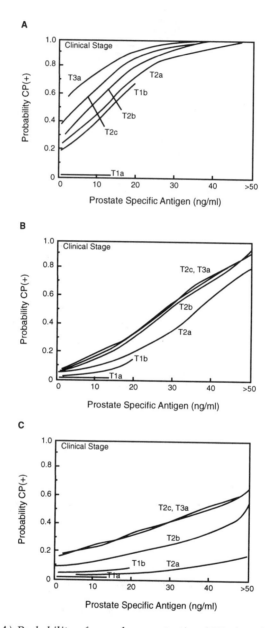

Fig. 7.4 *A) Probability of capsular penetration (CP+) as function of serum PSA and clinical stage by TNM classification system. B) Probability of seminal vesicle involvement (SV+) as function of serum PSA and clinical stage. C) Probability of lymph nodel involvement (LN+) as function of serum PSA and clinical stage.*

Table 7.3 *Distribution by pathologic stage of serum prostate-specific antigen (PSA) levels in men after radical prostatectomy*

PSA Level*	No. Men	No. (%) with OC	No. with CP	No. (%) with +SV/+LN
0–2.8	102	84 (82)	16 (16)	2 (2)
0–4	49	34 (69)	13 (27)	2 (4)
2.8–10	159	81 (51)	52 (33)	26 (16)
4–10	41	15 (37)	18 (44)	8 (20)
>4	40	23 (26)	26 (29)	47 (45)
>10	142	29 (20)	30 (21)	83 (59)
10–20	76	15 (20)	21 (28)	40 (52)
>20	62	14 (23)	7 (12)	41 (66)
20–50	43	11 (26)	4 (9)	28 (65)
>50	20	2 (10)	2 (10)	16 (80)
50–100	13	1 (8)	1 (8)	11 (84)
>100	6	0	0	6 (100)

*Tandem-R assay.
OC = organ-confined disease, CP = capsular perforation with or without positive margins, +SV = positive seminal vesicles, +LN = positive lymph nodes.
SOURCE: Reproduced with permission from Lange PH. Prostate-specific antigen for staging prior to surgery and for early detection of recurrence after surgery. Urol Clin North Am 1990;17:817.

ative pelvic CT scan or MRI is still being defined, and that these are not routinely performed by every urologist or at every hospital.

Radionuclide bone scans were traditionally obtained prior to surgery in all patients with prostate cancer. However, a study by Oesterling and colleagues (28) demonstrated that in 467 men who had a PSA of less than 8.0 mg/L, none had a positive bone scan. Therefore bone scans are no longer routinely obtained in men with PSA values of less than 8.0 mg/L prior to surgery.

■ PREOPERATIVE EVALUATION

Although some urologists (29) have advocated postponing surgery for 6 to 8 weeks following prostate needle biopsy and for 12 weeks following transurethral resection of the prostate, to avoid inflammatory adhesions or hematomas from distorting anatomic relationships near the prostate, we have found that a one-month interval is sufficient.

During this interval, we have the patient donate three units of autologous blood (one unit per week) prior to surgery. Ness and associates (30) showed no difference in the tumor recurrence rates in patients with prostate cancer who received autologous versus homologous blood. However, the use of autologous blood clearly eliminates the risk of transmission of infectious agents or transfusion reactions that may occur with homologous blood products.

Before surgery, the patient will require medical clearance from his internist, and he will we given an appointment to see the anesthesiologist. Patients are requested to avoid aspirin and nonsteroidal anti-inflammatory drugs for 10 days prior to surgery and while they are donating autologous blood. Most patients now are routinely admitted to the hospital on the morning of surgery.

■ SURGICAL TECHNIQUE

Radical Retropubic Prostatectomy

The radical retropubic prostatectomy was originally described by Millin (31) and modified by Campbell (32). However, in 1982 Walsh published a new technique, the so-called nerve-sparing radical retropubic prostatectomy (33). This technique was based on the identification of the neurovascular bundles that mediate erectile function. In the past decade and a half, this technique has emerged as the most popular approach for the surgical treatment of localized prostate cancer. However, it should be noted that this technique is also used even if the patient is impotent prior to surgery and when potency is not a postoperative concern. The so-called nerve-sparing radical retropubic prostatectomy is now more accurately called the anatomic radical retropubic prostatectomy. This is because the technique does much more than just attempt to preserve the nerves. Another important feature of this technique is the early identification and control of the dorsal venous complex. This potentially results in less blood loss and better identification of the anatomic structures during the surgery. Therefore, the terms *nerve-sparing radical retropubic prostatectomy* and *anatomic radical retropubic prostatectomy* are used interchangeably.

After adequate spinal, epidural, or general anaesthesia has been

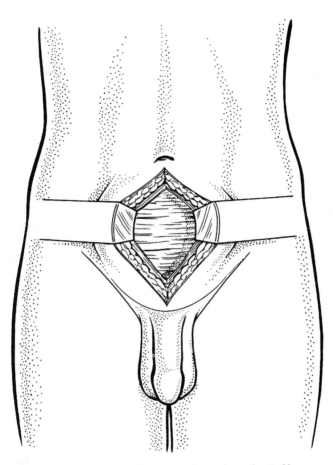

Fig. 7.5 *A midline infraumbical incision is made and a Balfour retractor is used for exposure.*

achieved, the patient is placed in the supine position. The midpoint between the umbilicus and the pubic symphysis is positioned over the break in the table. The table is maximally flexed, and the patient is placed in a mild Trendelenburg position. Our own preference is to place pneumatic boots that extend from the ankle to the thigh on the patient's legs, as a prophylaxis against deep venous thrombosis. A midline incision is made from the umbilicus to the symphysis pubis. The incision is carried down to the abdominal wall, and the space of Retzius is entered. A Balfour retractor is placed into the wound to facilitate exposure (Fig. 7.5). The external iliac veins are identified, and the overlying peritoneum is mobilized toward the head of the patient. The vasa deferentia are identified and divided between surgical clips. The malleable blade of the Balfour retractor is then placed to hold the bladder and the peritoneal contents in a cephalad direction. This exposure is necessary before starting the staging pelvic lymphadenectomy.

The areolar tissue overlying the external iliac vein is sharply excised. The overlying lymphatic tissue on the external iliac vein is cleaned off using sharp and blunt bisection. The lymphatics overlying the external iliac artery are preserved. The dissection proceeds inferiorly to the femoral canal, where surgical clips are used to ligate the lymphatic channels at the node of Cloquet. The obturator nodes are then removed, with special attention to avoid injury to the obturator nerve. It is usually not necessary to ligate the obturator artery and vein. The superior limit of the dissection is the bifurcation of the common iliac artery where the lymph nodes in the angle between the external iliac and hypogastric arteries are removed (Figs. 7.6). After a bilateral pelvic lymphadenectomy has been accomplished, attention is then turned to the radical prostatectomy.

The apical periprostatic fatty tissue is bluntly mobilized and excised. This maneuver exposes the endopelvic fascia. The endopel-

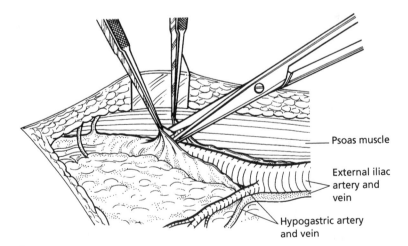

Psoas muscle

External iliac artery and vein

Hypogastric artery and vein

Fig. 7.6 *Lymphatic tissue is dissected off external iliac artery and vein.*

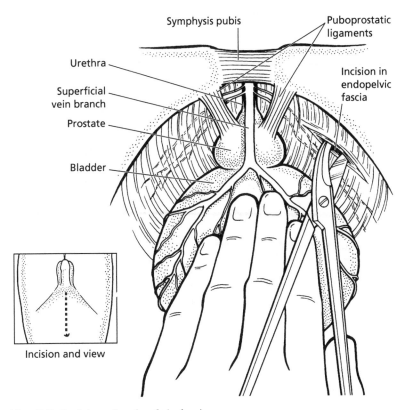

Fig. 7.7 *Incision of endopelvic fascia.*

vic fascia is sharply incised with the Metzenbaum scissors (Fig. 7.7). This fascia reflects over the obturator internus muscle. The endopelvic fascia is bluntly split to the level of the puboprostatic ligaments. The puboprostatic ligaments are then clearly seen and are sharply divided with scissors under direct vision (Fig. 7.8).

After division of the puboprostatic ligaments, the dorsal venous complex is clearly identified. The plane between the dorsal venous complex and the urethra can usually be palpated. The plane between the dorsal venous complex and the urethra is perforated with a right-angle clamp (Fig. 7.9). The right-angle clamp is spread in order to develop an adequate plane between the dorsal venous complex and the urethra. A number 0 silk suture is placed into the jaws of the

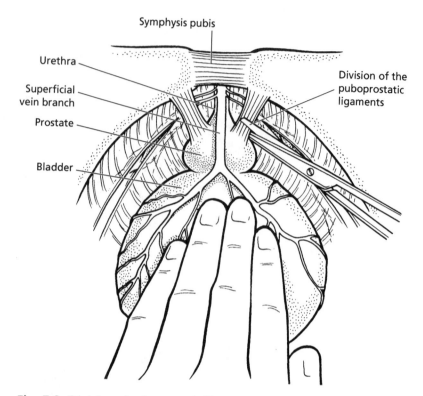

Fig. 7.8 *Division of puboprostatic ligaments.*

right-angle clamp with a suture passer (34) (Fig. 7.10). The right-angle clamp is then brought out and the 0 silk suture is tied down distally over the dorsal venous complex. This maneuver is performed a second time, and the 0 silk suture is tied proximally toward the apex of the prostate. Metzenbaum scissors are then used to divide the dorsal venous complex between the two silk ties. Occasionally after the division of the dorsal venous complex some bleeding continues from the dorsal vein stump. This is usually easily controlled with additional suture ligatures.

After division of the dorsal venous complex, the urethra comes clearly into view. The urethral catheter can easily be palpated within the urethra. Metzenbaum scissors are used to develop the plane between the urethra and the neurovascular bundles. The scissors are then used to divide the anterior wall of the urethra. The urethral

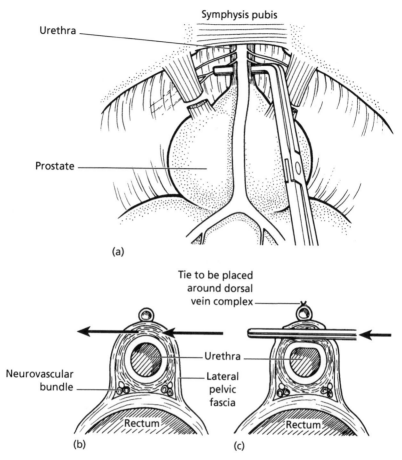

Fig. 7.9 *Right angle clamp is placed beneath dorsal vein complex.*

catheter then comes into view and a right-angle clamp is placed beneath the urethral catheter to bring it up into the field. A Kelly clamp is placed on the urethral catheter, and the urethral catheter is divided distal to the Kelly clamp. This enables the surgeon to keep the urethral catheter balloon inflated within the lumen of the bladder. The urethral catheter stump can then be used to provide traction to bring the prostate up into the surgical field. The posterior urethral wall is then divided. Metzenbaum scissors are then used to spread the rectourethralis muscle, and blunt finger dissection is used to develop the plane between the prostate and the anterior rectal wall.

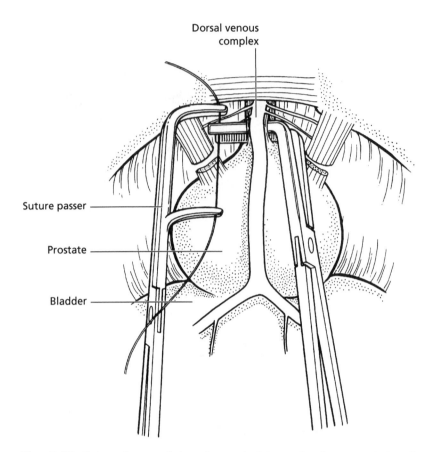

Dorsal venous
complex

Suture passer

Prostate

Bladder

Fig. 7.10 *Suture is passed into jaws of right-angle clamp, and dorsal venous complex is then ligated.*

At this point, the surgeon commences division of the lateral pelvic fascia and vascular pedicles. The neurovascular bundles are lateral and inferior to the lateral pelvic fascia, and they are swept away from the dissection to prevent injury (Fig. 7.11). As this dissection progresses, the anesthesiologist is asked to administer one ampule of indigo carmine intravenously to the patient. The indigo carmine will be excreted into the urine and will aid in the identification of the ureteral orifices later during the procedure.

As the lateral pelvic fascia is divided, the prostate is retracted cephalad, and this aids in the exposure of Denonvilliers' fascia. This fascia overlies the ampullae of the vasa deferentia and the seminal

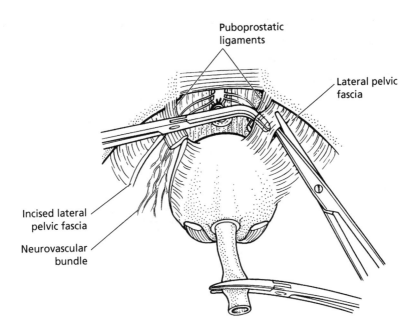

Fig. 7.11 *Division of lateral vascular pedicle.*

vesicles. Denonvilliers' fascia is sharply incised, and the ampullae of the vasa deferentia are exposed. A surgical clip is placed on each of the two ampullae and the ampullae are sharply divided. The residual lateral pedicle overlying the seminal vesicles is divided between surgical clips or suture ligatures. This maneuver helps to expose the seminal vesicles laterally.

Attention is now turned to the prostatovesicle junction. Traction on the Foley catheter facilitates identification of the bladder neck. It is often helpful to place some 0 chromic suture ligatures around some of the superficial veins that are on the anterior surface of the prostate. This will prevent back bleeding during division of the prostatovesicle junction. In addition, a stay suture is placed in the midline of the anterior bladder wall about 3 cm cephalad to the prostatovesicle junction, to provide traction during division of the bladder neck. The bladder neck is divided with cautery, and the Foley balloon can be seen in the bladder lumen. Indigo carmine–tinged urine is suctioned from the field. The bladder neck is divided laterally, and the ureteral orifices are identified. It is often useful to place 5F infant feeding tubes into the ureteral orifices to aid in their identification during division of the posterior bladder neck. After the posterior bladder neck has been successfully divided, the seminal vesicles are clearly in view. The seminal vesicles are each then dissected out to their distal tips. The arterial supply to the seminal vesicles is divided above surgical clips, and the surgical specimen is removed (Fig. 7.12).

The capacious bladder neck is then reconstructed to approach a diameter approximately the size of the pinky finger. The so-called tennis racquet technique for bladder neck closure is used. Interrupted 2-0 chromic catgut sutures are used to close the inferior portion of the bladder neck (Fig. 7.13). After the bladder neck has been closed to the proper diameter, the mucosa is everted outward with 4-0 chromic

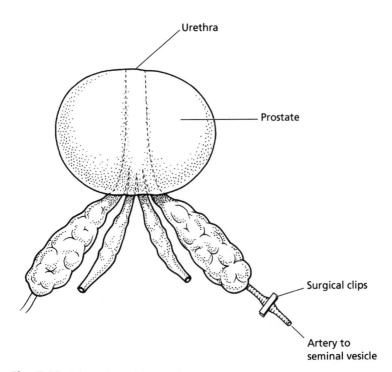

Fig. 7.12 *Dissection of seminal vesicles.*

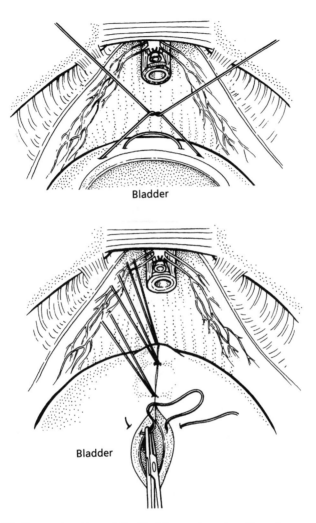

Fig. 7.13 *Reconstruction of the bladder neck, using "tennis-racquet" closure.*

catgut sutures to provide a mucosa-to-mucosa anastomosis and decrease the likelihood of postoperative bladder neck contracture.

The vesicourethral anastomosis is now performed. A 20 French 5-cc Foley balloon catheter is inserted through the urethra. Four to six absorbable sutures are placed through the distal urethral stump. Preference for the suture material differs from surgeon to surgeon, but all surgeons will use an absorbable suture of some type. Our own preference has been for 2-0 monocryl (Ethicon) suture material (Ethicon Endo-Surgery Inc., Cincinnati, Ohio). After the sutures have been placed in the urethral stump, the other ends of the sutures are placed through the reconstructed bladder neck. After all of the sutures have been placed, the old Foley catheter is removed and a new Foley catheter is inserted through the urethra and up through the bladder neck into the bladder lumen. The balloon is inflated to approximately 8 cc, and this is used to provide some traction on the bladder neck down toward the urethral stump. The anastomotic sutures are then tied down. After the anastomosis has been completed, the urethral catheter is irrigated with sterile saline to check for any leaks. The urethral catheter is then connected to a drainage bag. A Jackson-Pratt closed suction drain is placed in the pelvis and brought out through the skin through a separate stab wound incision. The abdominal incision is closed in the standard fashion.

Radical Perineal Prostatectomy

The radical perineal prostatectomy is another surgical alternative for the treatment of localized prostate cancer. Traditionally its main advantage has been less postoperative pain as compared with the radical retropubic prostatectomy. Its drawback has been the inability to perform a staging pelvic lymphadenectomy through the same incision. The decision as to whether to use a radical retropubic approach or a radical perineal approach is very much dependent on the surgeon's individual experience.

To perform a radical perineal prostatectomy, the sacrum is placed on the edge of the table and the buttocks are extended several inches over the edge of the table, with the legs padded and secured to stirrups (Fig. 7.14). Padded shoulder braces must also be used to prevent stretch or pressure injuries to the brachial plexus.

The Lowsley prostatic tractor is placed through the urethra and into the bladder, where the blades are opened. The skin incision is made anterior to the anal verge, and it is curved posterolaterally on either side within the medial borders of the ischial tuberosities. The superficial perineal fascia is incised with cautery, and the plane within the ischial rectal fossa is developed. The central tendon, which is the muscular sheath that extends anterior to the rectum, is also

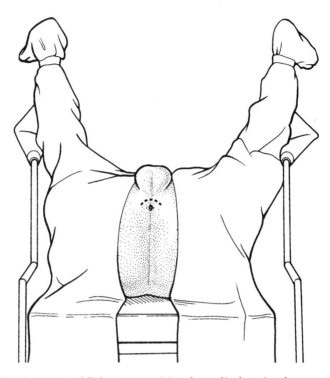

Fig. 7.14 *Exaggerated lithotomy position for radical perineal prostatectomy.*

divided with cautery (Fig. 7.15). The rectal sphincter is then visualized as an arch overlying the rectum. With blunt dissection, the rectum can be mobilized on either side of the rectourethralis muscle. The rectum is tented upward by the rectourethralis muscle, which is then divided, providing posterior displacement of the rectum. Blunt dissection continues, and this provides exposure of the lateral and anterior margins of the prostate. The fascia overlying the prostate should be white and glistening and is often referred to as "the pearly gates" (35,36) (Fig. 7.16).

The next maneuver is to expose the membranous urethra at the prostatic apex. A curved clamp is used to isolate the membranous urethra distal to the prostatic apex. The Lowsley tractor is then removed and the urethra is divided. A Young prostatic tractor is then passed through the prostatic urethra into the bladder, and the blades are opened. A plane is developed beneath the venous plexus, in

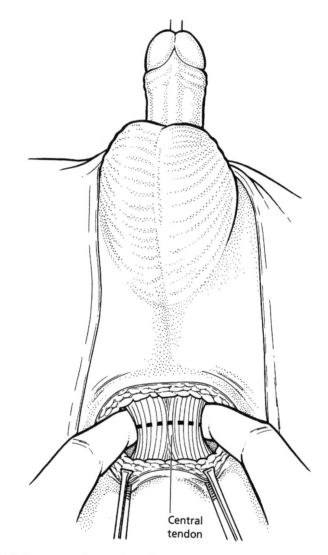

Fig. 7.15 *Exposure of central tendon.*

between the bladder and the prostate anteriorly. The prostate is then dissected off the bladder neck anteriorly. The bladder neck is then divided. At this point, the Young tractor can be withdrawn and a Foley catheter can be placed through the prostatic urethra and brought out through the line of incision between the prostate and the

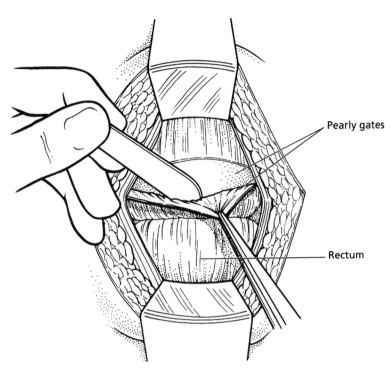

Fig. 7.16 *"Pearly gates" visualized.*

bladder neck. Traction on the catheter facilitates displacement of the prostate posteriorly and helps to define the plane between the bladder neck and the prostate. After the posterior bladder neck has been divided, the bladder is retracted upward and a plane is developed between the bladder anteriorly and the prostate and seminal vesicles posteriorly (Fig. 7.17). The vascular pedicles can be identified at five and seven o'clock and can be controlled with surgical clips or suture ligatures. After the vascular pedicles have been divided bilaterally, the specimen is held only by the seminal vesicles and vasa deferentia. The vasa are clipped and divided. The seminal vesicles are dissected out to their tips, and surgical clips are used to control their vascular supply. After the vascular supply to the seminal vesicles has been divided, the specimen is removed. The operative field is checked for hemostasis.

The bladder neck is then reconstructed in a similar manner as to

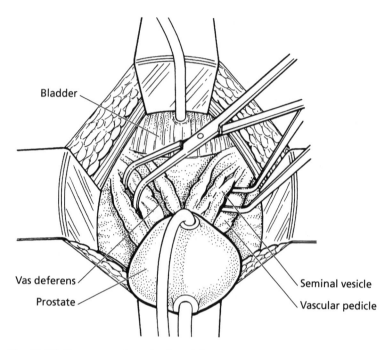

Fig. 7.17 *Exposure of seminal vesicles.*

that performed after a radical retropubic prostatectomy. The bladder neck is reconstructed so that its diameter is approximately that of a pinky finger. The bladder neck mucosa is everted with 4-0 chromic sutures, as after a radical retropubic prostatectomy. The anastomosis between the bladder neck and the urethral stump is then performed with 4-6 absorbable sutures. After the anastomosis is completed, a Penrose drain is brought out through a separate stab wound. The incision is closed in the usual manner. Levator ani muscles are approximated in the midline.

■ INTRAOPERATIVE COMPLICATIONS

Bleeding

The blood loss during a radical retropubic prostatectomy typically amounts to around 1,500 mL (three units of blood) (37,38). There has been some controversy in the literature as to whether intraoperative clamping of the hypogastric arteries diminishes blood loss. Peters and Walsh (37) reported a decease of transfusion requirements from 3.5 units per patient to 1.8 units per patient with intraoperative hypogastric artery clamping. However, Kavoussi and colleagues (38) found an average blood loss of 1,420 mL with hypogastric occlusion compared with 1,605 mL without hypogastric occlusion, and this difference was not statistically significant. Although no definitive resolution to this question has been reached, most urologists do not routinely clamp the hypogastric arteries intraoperatively during a radical retropubic prostatectomy.

There are three options for replacing blood lost intraoperatively: 1) homologous banked blood, 2) autologous blood donated prior to surgery, and 3) intraoperative mechanical autotransfusion (Cell-Saver Haemonetics Inc., Braintree, Massachusetts). All three methods have potential risks and benefits. Homologous banked blood has been used for decades to replace surgical blood loss. The potential risks include transmission of infectious agents (hepatitis, human immunodeficiency virus) and transfusion reactions. The benefits include enabling the patient to enter surgery with a normal hematocrit. Autologous blood transfusion requires the patient to donate one unit of blood per week for three weeks prior to surgery. This will render most patients slightly anemic at the time of surgery, but it eliminates the potential infectious complications of blood transfusion. As has been mentioned previously, Ness and colleagues (30) demonstrated no difference in prostate cancer recurrence whether the patient received autologous or homologous blood. With the third option, intraoperative mechanical autotransfusion devices are used to suction blood from the surgical field, remove debris, and retransfuse the blood back into the patient. Although these devices have never been clearly shown to increase the risk of recurrent cancer, there are at least theoretical concerns. First, work from our own laboratory has demonstrated that cells from several human tumor cell lines can survive passage through mechanical autotransfusion devices (39). Recent work by Libertino and colleagues (40) has demonstrated increased levels of PSA as measured by reverse transcriptase-polymerase chain reaction (RT-PCR) after dissection of the prostate during radical prostatectomy. Although there has been no clinical evidence that mechanical autotransfusions increase the risk of tumor recurrence after urologic surgery (41,42), it would appear prudent not to use these devices during radical prostatectomy unless absolutely necessary.

In addition to intraoperative bleeding, a small percentage of patients bleed postoperatively. Hedican and Walsh (43) reported that 7 of 1,350 consecutive radical prostatectomy patients developed significant enough postoperative bleeding to require blood transfusions. Their recommendation was that patients did better (fewer hospital days, lower risk of bladder neck contracture) if they were re-explored rather than managed conservatively.

Rectal Injury

Fortunately, rectal injury is also an uncommon event during radical prostatectomy. A rectal injury can occur whether the retropubic or the perineal approach is used; Borland and Walsh (44) reported a 1.0% rectal injury rate in 1,000 men undergoing radical retropubic prostatectomy. Rectal injuries should be closed with two layers of nonabsorbable sutures. Borland and Walsh recommended that omentum be interposed between the rectum and urethrovesical anastomosis (44). They also suggested that a diverting colostomy was not necessary to manage a rectal injury associated with a radical prostatectomy. However, many surgeons would prefer to perform a diverting colostomy if a rectal injury occurs.

■ POSTOPERATIVE CARE

Following surgery, the typical patient spends several hours in the recovery room and arrives in his hospital room by late afternoon. The optimal prophylaxis to prevent deep venous thrombosis and thromboembolism following surgery remains controversial (45). Walsh reported a 1.1% thromboembolic complication rate in a series of 900 radical retropubic prostatectomy patients (29). Others have reported deep vein thrombosis rates of 0.4% to 2.7% and a fatal pulmonary embolism rate of 0.6% (46–49). Our own practice has been to use pneumatic stockings intraoperatively and postoperatively in the hospital. The patient is also anticoagulated systemically with sodium warfarin (Coumadin) while he is in the hospital. However, it should be emphasized that the optimal method and duration of prophylaxis against thromboembolism following radical prostatectomy has not been established and will vary from surgeon to surgeon and from institution to institution.

The patient remains hospitalized until he is ambulating well and tolerating a full diet. The duration of hospitalization following radical prostatectomy is decreasing. Koch and Smith (50) recently reported a decrease at their institution from 5.8 hospital days prior to July 1993 to 3.5 hospital days since that time for patients undergoing radical prostatectomy. The urethral catheter remains in place following hospital discharge and is removed in the physician's office two to three weeks after surgery.

■ POSTOPERATIVE COMPLICATIONS

Impotence

Although the nerve-sparing radical prostatectomy is designed to preserve potency, impotence does occur following surgery. Walsh and Schlegel (51) first reported a 74% potency rate in 320 men followed for one to five years after nerve-sparing radical prostatectomy. A later report by Quinlan and colleagues (52) identified three factors that were correlated with the return of sexual function: 1) age, 2) clinical and pathologic stage, and 3) surgical technique (preservation or excision of the neurovascular bundle). They reported an overall potency rate of 68% postoperatively in men who were potent prior to surgery. They also stratified patients according to whether one or both neurovascular bundles had been preserved during surgery. In men under 50 years of age, the potency rate was similar whether a single or both neurovascular bundles had been preserved (90%). However, in men over the age of 50, there was a potency advantage in the group of patients who had both neurovascular bundles preserved.

Walsh (53) has further reported an overall potency rate of 72% among patients with stage A or B disease. Of those patients who regained their potency, it was recovered within 6 months in 59% of cases, one year in 95% of cases, 18 months in 99% of cases, and two years in 100% of cases. Walsh again reiterated the correlation between potency and patient age and tumor stage.

Not all investigators have equaled the potency rates of Walsh. Catalona (54) and Bigg, Kavoussi, and Catalona (55) have reported a potency rate of 63% in patients with bilateral nerve-sparing operations and 39% in those who had unilateral nerve-sparing procedures performed. However, Catalona's series differed from Walsh's, as the follow-up time was shorter and the patients were older with a generally higher stage of prostate cancer. At the present time, it is the practice of most urologists to perform bilateral nerve-sparing procedures whenever possible. However, cancer cure—not potency preservation—is the primary goal of the procedure. If there is evidence of extension of the tumor beyond the prostatic capsule, most surgeons will sacrifice one or both neurovascular bundles to achieve the best chance of cancer eradication.

Incontinence

Urinary incontinence will occur in some patients following radical prostatectomy. It is difficult to interpret much of the literature on postprostatectomy incontinence because the definitions of incontinence vary from report to report.

Ramon and colleagues (56) reported on 484 men who underwent radical retropubic prostatectomy for prostatic cancer. At six months postoperatively, 90% of the men were totally dry and 10% had stress incontinence. Pathologic stage and preservation of the neurovascular bundles had no influence on continence rates. They did observe that return to continence occurred sooner in men under the age of 70.

Steiner and colleagues (57) reported on a series of 593 consecutive patients who underwent an anatomic or nerve-sparing radical prostatectomy. Of these, 547 (92%) had total urinary control, 46 (8%) had stress incontinence, and 2 (0.3%) required the placement of an artificial urinary sphincter.

We examined the issue of incontinence following radical prostatectomy through a blind patient questionnaire (58). Of 196 patients who returned the questionnaire, 39 (20%) felt their postoperative urinary continence was excellent (the same as before surgery), 80 (41%) reported their continence as good (they needed no pads or external appliances), 61 (31%) stated their urinary control was fair (they wore pads or some type of external appliance but were not limited in terms of social activity), and 16 (8%) reported their urinary control was poor (they experienced continuous leaking). Only 3 patients (1.5%) required subsequent anti-incontinence surgery. Overall, only 10 patients (5%) said they would not undergo the surgery again. It is also important to note that patients reported that the time to their return to continence ranged from two weeks to two years.

Bladder Neck Contracture

It has been estimated that bladder neck contracture will occur in 3% to 12% of patients who undergo radical prostatectomy (29). Utilizing the technique popularized by Walsh (29), of everting the mucosa at the bladder neck, the incidence of bladder neck contracture should be minimized. Levy and colleagues (59) examined the impact of postoperative urinary extravasation at the anastomosis site and found no correlation between extravasation and subsequent bladder neck contracture.

When bladder neck contractures do occur, they will need to be periodically dilated. There is some concern that dilation of the bladder neck may diminish urinary continence, although in most cases this does not occur.

■ CONCLUSIONS

Radical prostatectomy, whether by the retropubic or perineal approach, is the cornerstone of surgical treatment for localized prostate cancer. It offers cancer cure rates superior to any other modality, and the complications can be managed successfully in the great majority of patients. Further refinements of technique will undoubtedly occur as urologists strive to maximize the efficacy of the procedure.

Editorial Comment

Like Odysseus, who was forced to navigate the narrow channel between Scylla and Charybdis—the twin monstrous rocks that threatened doom—the modern prostate cancer surgeon must perform his surgical dissection precisely. If the dissection is performed too far outside the prostatic capsule, there is a significant risk of damage to the neurovascular bundles, the urinary sphincter, or the rectum. If the dissection is too close to the prostate, there is a risk of cutting into the prostate and leaving prostate tissue and tumor, or of leaving microscopic extensions of malignant cells that extend past the prostatic capsule. Unlike Odysseus, however, it is not the surgeon who is in danger; it is the patient who risks impotence, urinary incontinence, or urethrorectal fistula and infection—or incomplete tumor resection and subsequent cancer growth.

There is no doubt that Walsh has contributed at least three technical innovations to radical prostatectomy: 1) early ligation of the dorsal vein complex with improved hemostasis so that the subsequent prostate dissection can be performed with better visualization in a less bloody field; 2) preservation of the neurovascular bundles with potential preservation of potency; and 3) a plane of dissection that hugs the prostatic capsule and makes damage to the urinary sphincter and possible incontinence, as well as rectal injury, less likely. These technical innovations have dovetailed with recent developments leading to earlier diagnosis of prostate cancer, so that now radical prostatectomy is more likely to be performed on patients with clinically early organ-confined disease.

A significant number of patients undergoing radical prostatectomy, however, have microextension (or gross extension) of tumor outside the prostate. The appropriate limits of dissection are not yet categorized well for these patients. In some patients neoadjuvant hormonal therapy is being used to shrink the tumor (and the prostate) prior to radical prostatectomy. The efficiency of this treatment and its potential technical benefits are controversial and remain unproven at the present time.

■ REFERENCES

1. Young HH. The cure of cancer of the prostate by radical perineal prostatectomy (prostato-seminal vesiculectomy): history, literature and statistics of Young's operation. J Urol 1995;53:188.
2. Marshall VF. Cancer of the prostate. In: Textbook of urology. New York: Paul B. Hoeber, 1956:213.
3. Millin T. Retropubic prostatectomy: new extravesical technique: report on 20 cases. Cancer 1945;2:693.
4. Memmelaar J. Total prostatovesiculectomy: retropubic approach. J Urol 1949;62:340.

5. Lattimer JK, Dean AL, Veenema R, Rafferty E. Radical prostatectomy for cancer. JAMA 1953;153:1347.

6. Chute R. Radical retropubic prostatectomy for cancer. J Urol 1954;71:347.

7. Walsh PC, Lepor H, Eggleston JC. Radical prostatectomy with preservation of sexual function: anatomical and pathological considerations. Prostate 1983;4:473.

8. Goluboff ET, Olsson CA. Urologists on a tightrope: Coping with a changing economy. J Urol 1994;151:1.

9. McLaughlin AP III. Radical retropubic prostatectomy. In: Harrison JH, Gittes RF, Perlmutter AD, et al. Campbell's urology. 4th ed. Philadelphia: WB Saunders, 1979:2315.

10. Middleton RG, Larsen RH. Selection of patients with stage B prostate cancer for radical prostatectomy. Urol Clin North Am 1990;17:779.

11. Frydenberg M, Oesterling JE. Therapeutic strategies for clinical stage C prostate cancer. In: Lange PH, guest ed. Problems in urology: therapeutic strategies in prostate cancer. Philadelphia: JB Lippincott, 1993;7:166.

12. Schroeder FH, Belt E. Carcinoma of the prostate: a study of 213 patients with stage C tumors treated by total perineal prostatectomy. J Urol 1975;114:257.

13. Zincke H, Utz DC, Benson RC Jr, Patterson DE. Bilateral pelvic lymphadenectomy and radical retropubic prostatectomy for stage C adenocarcinoma of prostate. Urology 1984;24:532.

14. Tomlinson RL, Currie DP, Boyce WH. Radical prostatectomy: palliation for stage C carcinoma of the prostate. J Urol 1977;117:85.

15. Middleton RG, Smith JA Jr, Melzer RB, Hamilton PE. Patient survival and local recurrence rate following radical prostatectomy for prostatic carcinoma. J Urol 1986;136:422.

16. Austenfeld MS, Davis BE. New concepts in the treatment of stage D-1 adenocarcinoma of the prostate. Urol Clin North Am 1990;17:867.

17. Kramer SA, Clone WA Jr, Farnham R, et al. Prognosis of patients with stage D1 prostatic adenocarcinoma. J Urol 1981;125:817.

18. Utz DC. Radical excision of adenocarcimoma of prostate with pelvic lymph node involvement: surgical gesture or curative procedure? Urology 1984;24(suppl):4.

19. Myers RP, Therneau TM, Zincke H, et al. Radical prostatectomy and the influence of early endocrine therapy for stage D1 prostate cancer: long-term follow up study. In: Multidisciplinary analysis of controversies in the management of prostate cancer. New York: Plenum Press, 1988:183.

20. Zincke H. Extended experience with surgical treatment of stage D1 adenocarcinoma of prostate. Urology 1989;33:27.

21. Catalona WJ, Millin DR, Kavoussi LR. Intermediate-term survival results in clinically under-staged prostate cancer patients following radical prostatectomy. J Urol 1988;140:540.

22. Oesterling JE, Chan DW, Epstein JI, et al. Prostate specific antigen in the preoperative and postoperative evaluation of localized prostatic cancer treated with radical prostatectomy. J Urol 1988;139:766.

23. Hudson MA, Bahnson RR, Catalona WJ. Clinical use of prostate specific antigen in patients with prostate cancer. J Urol 1989;142:1011.

24. Lange PH. Prostate-specific antigen for staging prior to surgery and for early detection of recurrence after surgery. Urol Clin North Am 1990;17:813.

25. Partin AW, Yoo J, Carter HB, et al. The use of prostate specific antigen, clinical stage and Gleason score to predict pathological stage in men with localized prostate cancer. J Urol 1993;150:110.

26. Lowe FC, Trauzzi SJ. Prostatic acid phosphatase in 1993: its limited clinical utility. Urol Clin North Am 1993;20:589.

27. Salo JO, Rannikko S. The value of acid phosphatase measurements in predicting extraprostatic cancer growth before radical prostatectomy. Br J Urol 1988;62:439.

28. Oesterling JE, Martin DK, Bergstralh EJ, Lowe FC. The use of prostate-specific antigen in staging patients with newly diagnosed prostate cancer. JAMA 1993;269:57.

29. Walsh PC. Radical retropubic prostatectomy. In: Walsh PC, Retik AB, Stamey TA, Vaughan ED Jr, eds. Campbell's urology. 6th ed. Philadelphia: WB Saunders, 1992:2865–2886.

30. Ness PM, Walsh PC, Zahurak M, et al. Prostate cancer recurrence in radical surgery patients receiving autologous or homologous blood. Transfusion 1992;32:31.

31. Millin T. Retropubic urinary surgery. Baltimore: Williams and Wilkins, 1947.

32. Campbell EW. Total prostatectomy with preliminary ligation of the vascular pedicle. J Urol 1959;81:464.

33. Walsh PC, Danker PF. Impotence following radical prostatectomy: insight into etiology and prevention. J Urol 1982;128:492.

34. Loughlin KR. Suture passer for pelvic and urological surgery. J Urol 1995;154:491.

35. Paulson DF. Technique of radical perineal prostatectomy. In: Skinner

DG, Lieskousky G, eds. Diagnosis and management of genitourinary cancer. Philadelphia: WB Saunders, 1987:721.

36. Paulson DR. Radical perineal prostatectomy. In: Lepor H, Lawson RK, eds. Prostate diseases. Philadelphia: WB Saunders, 1993:315.

37. Peters CA, Walsh PC. Blood transfusion and anesthetic practices in radical retropubic prostatectomy. J Urol 1985;134:81.

38. Kavoussi LR, Myers JA, Catalona WJ. Effect of temporary occlusion of hypogastric arteries on blood loss during radical retropubic prostatectomy. J Urol 1991;146:362–365.

39. Loughlin KR, Li H, Richmond G, et al. Preclinical assessment of human tumor cell depletion from peripheral blood lost during cancer surgery. Surgical Forum 1992;43:756.

40. Libertino JA, Vessella RL, Moisakis SC, et al. Detection and significance of circulating prostate cells using RT-PCR for messenger RNA PSA prior to and during radical prostatectomy. Presented at the New England Section of the American Urological Association meeting, Newport, Rhode Island, 1995. Abstract 14.

41. Klimberg I, Sirio R, Wajsman Z, Baker J. Intraoperative autotransfusion in urologic oncology. Arch Surg 1986;121:1326.

42. Hart OJ III, Klimberg I, Wajsman Z, Baker J. Intraoperative autotransfusion in radical cystectomy for carcinoma of the bladder. Surg Gynecol Obstet 1989;168:302.

43. Hedican SP, Walsh PC. Postoperative bleeding following radical retropubic prostatectomy. J Urol 1994;152:1181.

44. Borland RN, Walsh PC. The management of rectal injury during radical retropubic prostatectomy. J Urol 1992;147:905.

45. Kibel AS, Loughlin KR. Pathogenesis and prophylaxis of postoperative thromboembolic disease in urological pelvic surgery. J Urol 1995; 153:1763.

46. Igel RC, Barrett DM, Segura JW, et al. Perioperative and postoperative complications from bilateral pelvic lymphadenectomy and radical retropubic prostatectomy. J Urol 1987;137:1189.

47. Leandro P, Rossignol G, Gautier JR, Ramon J. Radical retropubic prostatectomy: morbidity and quality of life: experience with 620 consecutive cases. J Urol 1992;147:883.

48. Pedersen KV, Herder A. Radical retropubic prostatectomy for localized prostatic carcinoma: a clinical and pathological study of 201 cases. Scand J Urol Nephrol 1993;27:219.

49. Hautman RE, Sauter TW, Wenderoth UK. Radical retropubic

prostatectomy: morbidity and urinary continence in 418 consecutive cases. Urology 1994;43(suppl):47.

50. Koch MO, Smith JA. Cost containment in urology. Urology 1995;46:14.

51. Walsh PC, Schlegel PN. Radical pelvic surgery with preservation of sexual function. Ann Surg 1988;208:391.

52. Quinlan DM, Epstein JI, Carter BS, Walsh PC. Sexual function following radical prostatectomy: influence of preservation of neurovascular bundles. J Urol 1991;145:998.

53. Walsh PC. Radical prostatectomy, preservation of sexual function and cancer control: the controversy. Urol Clin North Am 1987;14:663.

54. Catalona WJ. Patient selection for results of and impact on tumor resection of potency-sparing radical prostatectomy. Urol Clin North Am 1990;17:819.

55. Bigg SW, Kavoussi LR, Catalona WF. Role of nerve-sparing radical prostatectomy for clinical stage B2 prostate cancer. J Urol 1990; 144:1420.

56. Ramon J, Leandro P, Rossignol G, Gartier JR. Urinary continence following radical retropubic prostatectomy. Br J Urol 1993;71:47.

57. Steiner MS, Morton RA, Walsh PC. Impact of anatomical radical prostatectomy on urinary continence. J Urol 1991;145:512.

58. Talcott JA, Richie JP, Loughlin KR. Incontinence following radical prostatectomy: assessment by patient survey. Presented at the American Urological Association meeting, San Antonio, Texas, 1993. Abstract 81.

59. Levy JBS, Ramchardani P, Berlin JW, et al. Vesicourethral healing following radical prostatectomy: is it related to surgical approach? Urology 1994;44:888.

Brachytherapy and Cryotherapy for Prostate Cancer

8

Anthony V. D'Amico
Kenneth I. Wishnow
Steven K. Clinton

■ **THE ROLE OF INTERSTITIAL RADIOTHERAPY IN THE MANAGEMENT OF CLINICAL ORGAN-CONFINED PROSTATE CANCER**

A renewed emphasis has been given to the use of interstitial brachytherapy as treatment for clinical organ-confined prostate cancer in selected patients. This interest has emerged because of advancements in the technical aspects of interstitial radiation delivery over the past five years and the ability to offer an expedient, cost-effective, and potentially less morbid treatment for early-stage carcinoma of the prostate. Specifically, computerized planning using computed tomography (1) or transrectal ultrasound (TRUS) guidance (2) have replaced "freehand" radioactive seed placement. Concurrent with these advances, techniques for prostate immobilization have also been developed (3). These modalities enhance the precision of radioactive seed loading, which improves the ability to achieve effective dosing of prostates varying in size and shape. A question remains, however: For whom does interstitial radioactive implantation offer optimal local control rates without undue risk of normal tissue morbidity?

Historical Perspective

The use of interstitial brachytherapy in the management of prostate cancer began in the 1960s under the direction of Scardino and Carlton at Baylor (4) and was developed later in the 1970s by Hilaris and Whitmore at the Memorial Sloan-Kettering Cancer Center (5). Their studies employed intraoperative retropubic placement of the I-125 implant using a freehand technique. Three institutions (6–8) have reported a retrospective analysis of clinical local control with freehand-placed interstitial radioactive seeds versus external beam radiation therapy, stratified by clinical stage (Table 8.1). Clinical local control was significantly less for patients with stage B and C lesions having implant therapy, compared with external beam radiation. Moreover, Kuban and colleagues (7) found that major complications, attributable to local recurrence, were more frequent in implanted patients compared with those receiving external beam therapy (20% versus 8%; $p = 0.006$).

It was speculated (8) that an inhomogeneous dose distribution, due to the geometrically unacceptable radioactive seed placement

Table 8.1 *Clinical local failure rates for freehand I-125 prostatic implantation and external beam radiation therapy*

Investigator (Institution)	Stage A2		Stage B		Stage C	
	Implant	External Beam	Implant	External Beam	Implant	External Beam
Koprowski et al. (6) (Hahnemann)[a]	6%	0%	52%	6%	67%	17%
Kuban et al. (7) (Eastern Virginia Medical School)[b]	9%	3%	26%	13%	44%	26%
Morton and Peschel (8) (Yale)[c]	0%	0%	17%	4%	29%	18%

[a] 5-year absolute values; 101 patients with implants, with median follow-up of 57 mo; 175 with external beam radiation therapy, with median follow-up of 67 mo. Local failure defined by (DRE) only.
[b] 10-year absolute values; 120 patients with implants and 246 with external beam radiation therapy, with median follow-up of 80 mo. Local failure defined by DRE and biopsy when exam was equivocal.
[c] 10-year absolute values; 147 patients with implants and 166 with external beam radiation therapy, median follow-up not stated. Local failure defined by DRE; proven by biopsy.

achieved with the freehand technique, led to underdosing of tumor. This resulted in decreased local control when compared with external beam radiation therapy, which by design has dose homogeneity across the entire prostate. Conversely, localized areas of high dose within, or adjacent to, the prostate, arising from seeds clustered near vital structures (urethra, rectum, bladder, periprostatic neurovascular tissue), could have contributed to the high frequency of urethral stenosis, incontinence, rectal ulceration, and prostatic-rectal fistula.

Modern Techniques

Transrectal Ultrasound-Guided Transperineal Implant: The first method employed for both the preoperative calculation of the optimal radioactive seed arrangement and the intraoperative seed localization was transrectal ultrasound (2), and it is depicted in Figure 8.1. Using a TRUS probe, the prostatic capsule is outlined on each image, obtained at 5mm intervals on 5-mm-thick slices from the apex to the

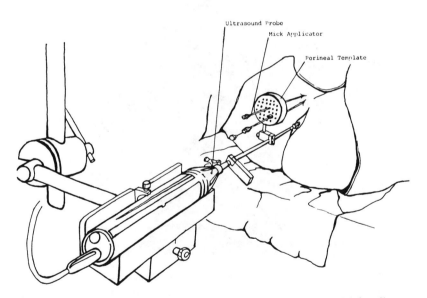

Fig. 8.1 *Transrectal ultrasound-guided transperineal interstitial radiotherapy. The apparatus includes the perineal template, ultrasound probe, and MICK applicator (9). (Reproduced by permission from Priestly JB. Use of MICK applicator in transperineal ultrasound-guided ^{125}I seed implantation. J Endourol 1990;4:375–379.)*

base of the gland. A computerized algorithm is used to calculate the optimal seed distribution that can be achieved using a transperineal approach in conjunction with a template grid directed over the prostate. This technique allows the clinician to deliver an adequate dose to the entire target volume, which is assumed to be equal to the ultrasound-derived prostate volume. Intraoperatively, the needle-guide template is mounted against the perineum, and up to three needles not containing radioactive seeds are initially inserted for immobilization of the prostate. The ultrasound probe is placed to correspond to the level of the prostate base, and an approximation of the maximal depth to which the needle should be inserted is gauged by visualizing when the needle comes into view on the ultrasound screen (Fig. 8.2A). This method provides only an approximation,

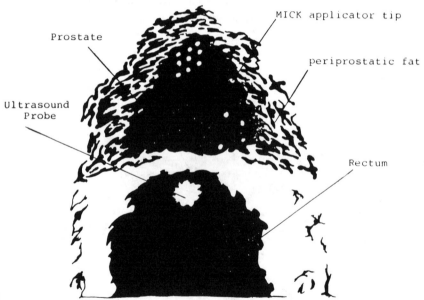

A

Fig. 8.2 *A) Ultrasound image of the prostate showing the appearance of the tip of the MICK applicator and confirming localization of the seeds with respect to the prostatic capsule. B) Fluoroscopic anterior-posterior image allowing for intraoperative localization of the MICK applicator (9) with respect to the urethra (black arrow) and Foley balloon. C) Fluoroscopic lateral image allowing for intraoperative localization of the MICK applicator with respect to the urethra (black arrow) and Foley balloon.*

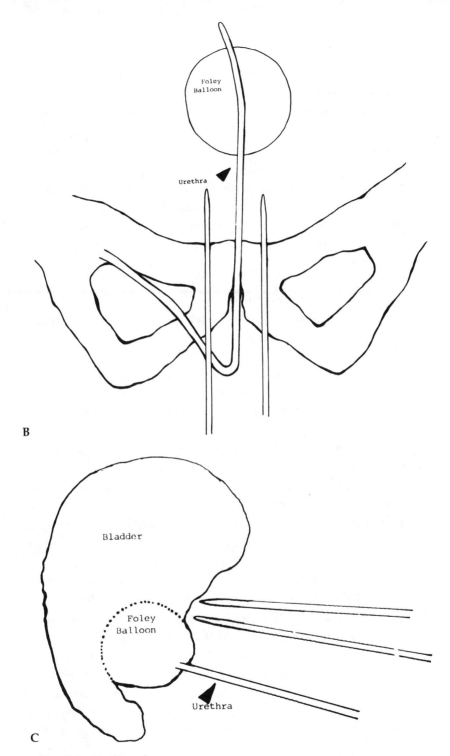

Fig. 8.2 *Continued*

because when the prostate is implanted, the base can be lifted 1 to 2 cm above its resting position. Therefore, more accurate methods for ensuring coverage of the prostatic base include: (a) radiopaque internal markers placed at the prostate base, (b) cystoscopic evaluation after implantation to ensure appropriate positioning into the prostatic base but not into the bladder, (c) placing the needles through the bladder and then retracting until the needles are in the prostatic base as verified by ultrasound. The seeds can then be deposited using a MICK applicator (9) or Mannen needles (10). A recent development that further enhances seed placement is a product called Rapid Strand (Medi-Physics, Amersham Healthcare, Arlington Heights, Illinois) in which the sources are affixed to a dense suture, which ensures fixed spacing between sources along the line of application.

CT-Directed Transperineal Implant: CT-based techniques (1) for both the localization of the prostate and for radioactive seed dosimetry have also been introduced. In an analogous manner to the TRUS technique, a preoperative planning CT is obtained using 5-mm slices, and the periphery of the prostate gland is carefully outlined. A radiopaque wire in the Foley catheter and contrast in the Foley balloon allow for visualization of the urethra on the planning CT scout image as well as during seed placement using fluoroscopy. Intraoperatively, the gland is immobilized in the same manner as described for the TRUS-directed technique, and the positions of the needles are checked by both anterior-posterior (Fig. 8.2B) and lateral (Fig. 8.2C) fluoroscopy to determine their correct position relative to the urethra. The needle depth is gauged by its spatial relationship to the inferior aspect of the Foley balloon on the anterior-posterior fluoroscopic view. Similar to the ultrasound technique, using the Foley balloon as a guide for the prostate base can result in an error of 1 to 2 cm because of prostate motion during implantation. Therefore, the methods described for localization of the prostate base in the ultrasound section, such as radiopaque markers or cystoscopic guidance, can also be used during fluoroscopy-directed placement of the radioactive seeds.

The major difference between the two approaches is the point of reference for prostate localization. With TRUS-based planning, the prostatic capsule is used to judge the correct placement of the radioactive seeds, whereas with CT-based planning, the contrast-filled urethra is used for reference. Both techniques require regional or general anesthesia.

Outcome of Implant, External Beam Radiation, and Radical Prostatectomy for Clinical Stage T1 and T2 Disease

Table 8.2 summarizes the three-year actuarial freedom from PSA failure and late complication rates for patients from several large implant (11–14), surgical (15–16), and external beam radiation series. The radiation series (17–24) report 80% to 94% three-year actuarial freedom from PSA failure rates with median follow-up ranging from 18 months to 7.8 years for all patients with clinical stage T1 and T2 disease. Likewise, the surgical series report 85% to 87% three-year actuarial freedom from PSA failure rates, with median follow-up ranging from 1.8 to 4.4 years in patients with clinical stage T1 and T2 disease. The three-year freedom from biochemical failure rates for implant patients from the Wallner (11), Priestly (12), and Russo (13) series are numerically lower, at 76% to 83%, than those reported from the external beam radiation and surgical series. The exception is the large and favorable cohort of patients treated by implant and reported by Blasko and colleagues (14). For the patients treated with an implant and who had an initial PSA less than 10 ng/mL, the three-year biochemical control rates are 87% to 96%, similar to those reported from the external beam and surgical series. However, it is important to note that this is a retrospective comparison and that the definition of biochemical failure varied between series, ranging from normalization of PSA (i.e., <4 ng/mL on the Hybritech scale) (11–14) to undetectable PSA (<0.2 ng/mL on the Hybritech scale) (15–16).

Three-year actuarial potency rates are comparable, ranging from 45% to 50% in the external beam radiation series, from 22% to 90% in the surgical series depending on age and the type of operation, and 50% to 81% (two-year actuarial) or 85% (three-year crude) in the implant series, depending on age at the time of treatment. It is important to note, however, that Bagshaw and colleagues (18) have previ-

Table 8.2 Three-year actuarial freedom from biochemical failure (FFBF) and late complications after transperineal interstitial radiation therapy, external beam radiation therapy, and radical prostatectomy for clinical stage T1 and T2 lesions

Treatment Modality	No. Patients	Clinical Stage (% T1:% T2)	Median Follow-up	Specific Patient Factors	3-yr FFBF Rate (PSA < 10)[a]	Potency Rate[b]	Late Complications GI	Late Complications GU
Implant								
Priestly and Beyer (12)	130[c]	5:95	max 2.3 yr	—	76% (87%)	90%[d]	NR	NR
Wallner et al. (11)	62	24:76	1.6 yr	—	83%	81%	13.0%[e]	10.0%[f]
Russo et al. (13)	51	NR	1.7 yr	Lap LN (−)	77% (96%)	NR	NR	NR
Blasko et al. (14)	197[g]		3.0 yr		93% (94%)	85%, 70%[h]	1.0%[i]	19.0%[i]
External Beam Radiation								
Bagshaw et al. (17,18)	377	33:67	7.8 yr	T1, T2a	90%[j]	50%	3.9%	4.4%
Hanks et al. (RTOG) (20)	104	15:85	9.4 yr	—	94%[j]	33%	11.5%	16.8%
Liebel et al. (3-D planning) (21)	324	15:53: 32(T3)	1.5 yr	PSA < 20, Gleason sum 6	96%	70%	4.3%	3.3%

Shipley et al. (22,23)	74	12:88	7.3 yr	PSA < 15, Gleason sum 6	83%[k]	45%	16.3%	17.3%
Zagars (24)	112	45:55	3.3 yr	Gleason sum 6	80%	NR	4.6%	5.3%
Surgery								
Catalona and Swith (15)	194	21:79	approx. 1.8 yr	Gleason sum 4	85% (95%)	52%	—	10.0%
Walsh et al. (16)	955	17:83	4.4 yr	—	87%	22%–90%[l]	—	8.0%

a Results in parentheses represent 3-yr FFBF for patients with initial PSA < 10 ng/mL.
b Evaluated at the time of median follow-up.
c Crude rate at 21 mo for 26 of the 130 treated patients available for follow-up.
d Crude potency rate; time at which value was measured and how potency was assessed not stated.
e Radiation Therapy Oncology Group, grade 2 rectal ulceration; two-fifths of patients with this complication required colostomy.
f Genitourinary complications requiring transurethral resection of prostate.
g Favorable cohort: PSA < 4 ng/mL (30%); biopsy Gleason sum 2–4 (53%); clinical stage T2a (89%).
h Crude potency rates were 85% (age <70) and 70% (age >70).
i Crude rates.
j Freedom from clinical failure, pathologically node negative.
k Reported in Shipley, Zietman, Hanks, et al. (22).
l Actuarial value as a function of age (<50 to >70).
NR = not reported.

ously reported on 434 initially potent patients treated with external beam radiation therapy at Stanford, finding a two-year actuarial potency preservation rate of 80% with a median follow-up of two years. Therefore, further follow-up is necessary to truly determine if interstitial radiotherapy maintains a potency advantage compared with external beam radiotherapy. Ideally, an assessment of potency after interstitial radiotherapy using the questionnaire developed by Talcott and colleagues (19) would allow a direct and independent comparison to the potency rates achieved after treatment with external beam radiation therapy or radical prostatectomy.

Short-term follow-up (19 months median) of the implant-treated patients revealed significant gastrointestinal and genitourinary complication rates: 12% and 10%, respectively (calculated actuarially at two years). These high complication rates, necessitating colostomy because of prostatic-rectal fistula, or transurethral resection of the prostate (TURP) for urinary continence, most likely are the result of a high dose of radiation delivered to the anterior rectal mucosa because of juxtaposed palpable disease, or to the urethra because of implant geometry.

Further follow-up will determine whether the implant-managed patients with a PSA level under 10 ng/mL maintain superior rates of potency preservation and equivalent rates of freedom from biochemical failure compared with those achieved using external beam radiation or radical prostatectomy. Late gastrointestinal and genitourinary grade 3 complications, however, are increased despite a median follow-up of less than two years in the Wallner (11) implant series and 37 months in the Blasko (14) series. The more recent experiences using newer techniques report a marked diminution in complications, and further follow-up of these more recent studies may illustrate PSA control with less morbidity.

Factors That Determine the Best Implant Candidates

It is interesting to note that even during the freehand era of prostate interstitial radiation therapy, local control appeared equivalent to external beam radiation therapy for stage A2 disease (6–8). In the Wallner study (11), using modern techniques, there were no failures in patients with nonpalpable (T1c, T1b) disease with a median follow-up of 19 months. The dosimetry of the implant and careful selection of appropriate implant candidates provides a possible explanation.

Prostate Cancer Location: The location of the cancer within the prostate gland is particularly relevant when treating with interstitial radiotherapy. Unlike external beam radiotherapy, where a homogenous dose distribution encompassing the entire prostate is readily achievable, the dose distribution resulting from the implant is directly related to the positioning of the radioactive seeds within the gland. The primary concern (unless differential loading of source activity is implemented) is that the geometry of the prostate gland necessitates high central doses to achieve a minimally effective peripheral dose. This is because the central dose is derived from both the centrally and peripherally located sources. In contrast, rapid dose falloff is seen in the outermost aspect of the peripheral zone, because the dose to the area is delivered primarily from peripheral sources and not peripheral plus central sources. Previous whole-mount studies (25) of radical prostatectomy specimens have shown that the majority of prostate cancers arise in the peripheral zone (68%), with a substantial minority originating in the periurethral transitional region (24%) and the least frequent location being the central zone (6%). Therefore, peripherally based tumors, which comprise the majority (approximately two-thirds) of all prostate cancers, are located in the region of the prostate receiving doses at, or slightly above, the minimum peripheral dose. Any further extension of tumor toward the prostatic capsule potentially allows the disease to exist in the region of rapid implant dose falloff.

The results of several investigations (25–27) examining pathologic features as a function of clinical stage are listed in Table 8.3. Epstein and colleagues (26) found that patients with clinical stage A1 (13%) or B (87%) prostate cancer had 8% and 66% extracapsular extension (ECE), respectively, while 3% and 43% had positive surgical margins (PSM). Rosen and colleagues (25) evaluated 144 prostatectomy specimens from clinical stage A (32%) and B (68%) patients and showed ECE in 22% and 63%, and PSM in 22% and 23%, respectively. D'Amico and associates (27) found 29% and 30% of patients

Table 8.3 *Extracapsular extension and positive surgical margin rates as function of clinical state*

	T1a,b	T2a,b,c
Extracapsular Extension		
Epstein et al. (26)	8%[a]	66%
Johns Hopkins		
Rosen et al. (25)	22%	63%
Baylor		
D'Amico et al. (27)	29%[b]	30%[c]
Penn		
Positive Surgical Margins		
Epstein et al. (26)	3%[a]	43%
Rosen et al. (25)	22%	23%
D'Amico et al. (27)	21%[b]	23%[c]

[a] T1a.
[b] T1a,b,c.
[c] T2a,b.

with clinical stage T1 and T2a,b, respectively, to have ECE. Similarly, 21% and 23% of clinical stage T1, T2a,b patients had PSM. Therefore, it appears that clinical stage T1 lesions are associated with 20% to 30% of patients exhibiting extracapsular extension and approximately 20% having positive surgical margins. Exceptions are T1a lesions, where both ECE and PSM are seen in fewer than 10% of patients. Likewise, for clinical stage T2a,b,c lesions it can be predicted that 30% to 60% of patients have ECE and 20% to 40% will have PSM.

Therefore, based on dosimetric considerations, the ideal implant candidate would be a patient with an intraprostatic primary tumor completely encompassed by the gland and therefore located within the adequate- to high-dose treatment volume. Patients with nonpalpable (T1c) tumors, whose risk of extraprostatic disease is minimal, may be the optimal implant candidates. As illustrated by the Wallner study (11), where at least 50% of all patients were at low to moderate risk for extraprostatic disease (PSA < 10 ng/mL and biopsy Gleason sum 2 to 7), none of the 13 patients with T1c disease experienced biochemical failure at a median follow-up of 19 months. Similarly, in the favorable cohort reported by Blasko and colleagues (14), none of the 34 T1c patients failed biochemically at a median follow-up of 37 months. In contrast, patients with a previous history of surgical manipulation of the urethra (e.g., TURP) have been shown to have an increased rate of late genitourinary complications, particularly incontinence (11,14).

Clinical Stage: Several investigators (26–29) have quantified the clinical and pathologic characteristics of T1c tumors (Table 8.4). In particular, Oesterling and colleagues (28) reported that 86% of T1c patients (n = 208) had the predominant location of tumor pathologically documented in the peripheral zone, analogous to what is observed for palpable lesions. Interestingly, Epstein and colleagues (29) found that the mean tumor volume of T1c lesions (n = 157) was not significantly different than that of palpable tumors. Yet, in both the Oesterling and Epstein series it was found that the mean gland size in patients harboring clinical stage T1c lesions was significantly larger ($p = 0.001$) than in those patients with clinically palpable organ-confined lesions. Epstein postulated that a larger gland volume may influence tumor palpability. If true, then a T1c lesion would satisfy at least some of the criteria for an ideal implant candidate, since at least the posterior and the posterolateral aspect of the gland, where palpation can be performed, is without evidence of extraprostatic disease.

Table 8.4 *Pathologic characteristics of clinical stage T1c prosate cancer*

Author	No. Patients	Organ-Confined	Extracapsular Extension	Positive Surgical Margins	Seminal Vesical Invasion
Epstein et al. (29) Johns Hopkins	157	51%	49%	17%	6%
Oesterling et al. (28) Mayo Clinic	208	53%	35%	34%	9%

Unfortunately, T1c lesions are not exclusively organ confined. Oesterling (28) found that only 53% were pathologically organ confined and that 35% had extracapsular extension, 9% had seminal vesicle invasion, and 66% had positive surgical margins that were comparable to clinical stage T2 lesions. Likewise, Epstein and colleagues in a separate analysis (29), found that 51% of clinical stage T1c patients were clinically organ confined, 15% had focal extracapsular extension, 34% had established extracapsular extension, 6% had seminal vesicle invasion, and 17% had positive surgical margins. Therefore, lack of a palpable lesion is not sufficient to define a tumor that is purely intraprostatic. Additional clinical factors, including PSA and the biopsy Gleason sum, have been shown to aid in selecting patients who have pathologic organ-confined disease.

Gleason Score and PSA: Partin and colleagues (30) found that the combination of the PSA, clinical stage, and biopsy Gleason sum were superior to any one of these indicators in predicting pathologic stage. Specifically, 82% of the subgroup having clinical stage T1c, a PSA under 10 ng/mL, and a Gleason sum of 2 to 4 had pathologic organ-confined disease at prostatectomy. This is a marked improvement over the 51% and 53% noted by Epstein and Oesterling, respectively, for all clinical stage T1c patients. Moreover, once the PSA is greater than 10 ng/mL, despite a biopsy Gleason sum of 2 to 4, fewer than 61% of patients showed organ-confined disease. Likewise, for a Gleason sum of 5 or more, even with a PSA under 10 ng/mL, no more than 71% of patients with T1c disease were found to have pathologic organ-confined disease. These results (Table 8.5) suggest that to have a minimal risk of extraprostatic disease, which extends beyond the high-dose implant volume, optimal candidates are those with a PSA under 10 ng/mL and a Gleason sum of 2 to 4 (31).

Conclusions

There has been a great deal of discussion in the recent medical literature and the popular press devoted to "seed implants" for the definitive treatment of clinically localized prostate cancer. The use of CT or TRUS for planning and templates for seed insertion rather than freehand implantation has improved the dosimetry. The short treatment

Table 8.5 *Pathologic organ-confined disease in clinical stage T1c patients as a function of the biopsy Gleason sum and prostate-specific antigen (PSA)*

Gleason Sum	PSA (ng/mL)	Pathologic Organ-Confined Disease
All T1c patients	All T1c patients	51%–53%
4	<10	82%
4	>10	61%
5	<10	71%

SOURCE: Reproduced by permission from Partin AW, Yoo J, Carter HB, et al. The use of prostate specific antigen, clinical stage and Gleason score to predict pathological stage in men with localized prostate cancer. J Urol 1993;150:110–114.

time, similar to surgery, involved with implant therapy is appealing to patients. However, the potential benefits must be placed in context with the risk of long-term toxicity. A review of the available literature suggests that a combination of clinical stage, PSA, and biopsy Gleason sum allow for the selection of patients who will have the highest probability of having all of the prostate cancer encompassed by the high-dose implant volume while simultaneously respecting the normal tissue tolerance doses of the juxtaposed tissues (rectum and bladder). In particular, patients with nonpalpable (T1c) lesions, a biopsy Gleason sum under 6 (ideally 4), and a PSA under 10 ng/mL represent the optimal implant candidates. Differential loading of the implants away from the center, and avoiding men who have large prostate glands (60 cc) or a history of TURP as implant candidates may reduce urethral complications. Further follow-up of men treated with interstitial radiotherapy will determine if potency preservation and freedom from biochemical failure are inferior, equivalent, or superior to radical prostatectomy or external beam radiation therapy for specific subgroups.

■ THE ROLE OF CRYOTHERAPY IN THE MANAGEMENT OF PROSTATE CANCER

Cryoablation of the prostate has reemerged in recent years as an alternative to radical prostatectomy or radiotherapy (either external beam or radioactive seed implantation) for treatment of localized prostate cancer. The current wave of interest in this procedure among the medical community is the result of the improved technology involved in visualization of the prostate, percutaneous instrumentation, and the cryotherapy delivery systems. In addition, patient interest has increased because of dissatisfaction with standard therapies.

Cryoablation is an invasive procedure that is performed under regional or general anesthesia in the operating room. The goal of cryoablation is destruction of the malignant and benign epithelium of the prostate by exposure to rapid freezing and thawing at extreme temperatures. Studies in the canine model show that the prostatic epithelium and stroma undergo hemorrhagic necrosis, similar to ischemic injury, while the architectural framework of the gland remains and undergoes a reepithelialization from a transitional cell epithelium progenitor (32). Since the mechanism of cell death is direct destruction of the tumor, radical surgery and cryotherapy share the same goals (complete elimination of the diseased prostatic epithelium) and the same limitations (failure to destroy malignant cells that have spread outside the borders of the prostate).

In the rush of excitement about this new technology, some enthusiasts have postulated that cryoablation can minimize destruction of adjacent normal tissue and thereby preserve urinary continence and sexual potency while also reliably destroying prostate cancers, including those that have spread through the prostatic capsule. Unfortunately, these claims may be unrealistic. The cryosurgical procedure is basically a cold-medium technology extension of the surgical knife. When it is used to aggressively destroy tissue outside the prostatic capsule, urinary incontinence, impotence, or rectal injury may ensue. When used timidly, there may be incomplete prostate tumor destruction and progressive cancer growth. The potential advantages are several. Cryotherapy may be delivered through thin probes that are placed percutaneously, sparing the patient a large surgical procedure. In addition, cryotherapy may be used repeatedly, in combination with, or following other therapies to treat prostate cancer. The potential disadvantage is that it may be very difficult to reliably freeze the entire prostate and kill all viable tumor cells, while avoiding significant damage to surrounding structures such as the urinary sphincters, neurovascular bundles, and rectum.

Historical Perspective

Cryoablation of the prostate was originally piloted in the canine model in 1964 (33). The initial application of this procedure in humans diagnosed with BPH or prostate cancer used a transurethral approach, with the cryoprobe blindly positioned using rectal palpation. Morbidity was high in these patients due to urethral sloughing of necrotic tissue, contributing to urinary outflow obstruction (34). In addition, the transurethral approach did not adequately treat the posterior peripheral zone of the prostate, where tumors are common. The more extensive freezing needed to reach these lesions contributed to higher rates of sloughing as well as injury to the bladder and bowel wall. Cryotherapy was further developed in the 1970s by Flocks and colleagues (35) with the introduction of the open perineal procedure, which improved visualization and allowed the cryoprobe to be placed directly into the malignant nodule. In 1982, Bonney reported 5- and 10-year follow-up data on 229 patients who had undergone open perineal cryosurgical ablation, with survival rates that were similar to stage-matched men undergoing radical prostatectomy (36). Although urethral sloughing was less frequent, local complications, such as urethrocutaneous and urethrorectal fistulas, were often the result of the open perineal approach. The inexact probe positioning and the inability to precisely monitor the freezing zone lead many to abandon this approach until modern ultrasound methods were applied in the late 1980s (37). The use of real-time TRUS allowed practitioners to precisely position the cryoprobe and regulate the freezing process using a closed percutaneous procedure (38,39). In addition, the risk of urethral sloughing can be further reduced by intraoperative urethral warming. The current technology is rapidly becoming available, and will increase patient satisfaction.

Modern Techniques

Cryoablation is performed in the operating room under regional or general anesthesia (40). With the patient in the lithotomy position, a suprapubic tube (necessary for post-treatment bladder drainage for 5 to 14 days) is placed, under cystoscopic visualization. A urethral catheter is placed to facilitate urethral visualization by TRUS as well as to circulate warm water to the urethra and bladder in order to minimize damage to these tissues during the freezing process. With careful monitoring by TRUS, up to five 3-mm-diameter cryoprobes are introduced percutaneously into the prostate through the perineum. The distal 4 cm of the cryoprobe induces freezing, and the iceball extends about 1 cm from the probe. Optimal placement of the probes allows the entire prostate gland and some extraprostatic tissue to be completely engulfed by the contiguous ice ball derived from the five probes. The skill of the operator is crucial to completely treat prostate glands of diverse size and shape without skipping areas, while simultaneously avoiding injury to important adjacent tissues. Freezing is accomplished by circulation through the cryoprobes of liquid nitrogen at −180 to −200 degrees centigrade. Careful monitoring of the freezing process is provided by TRUS, and one or two freeze-thaw cycles may be used. The dosimetry at the edges of the ice ball are poorly understood, and the number of cycles of freezing and thawing that are optimal for maximal tumor cell kill are unknown.

The usual hospital stay is one to two days. Most patients experience gross hematuria, some degree of perineal and scrotal swelling, and ecchymosis during the first 24 hours. The suprapubic tube is used to drain the bladder until adequate spontaneous voiding through the urethra occurs 5 to 14 days after the procedure. Follow-up care should include inquiry into complications such as sexual dysfunction and incontinence, serial PSA, digital rectal examinations, and TRUS. Sextant biopsies using TRUS after several months may provide the best assessment of residual viable tumor cells. Repeat cryotherapy could be performed if residual tumor is noted, or the patient may proceed to other forms of therapy.

Outcomes of Cryotherapy for Prostate Cancer

The earliest data concerning ultrasound-guided perineal cryotherapy as the primary treatment for clinically localized prostate cancer described the application of modern technology with minimal short-term morbidity (39). A subsequent report described 62 patients with stage C prostate cancer who averaged one year of follow-up (41). These patients received postcryotherapy biopsies at three months, as well as serial PSA determinations. At three months, 49 of 52 patients (79%) had negative biopsies. The median PSA for the patients with negative biopsies was 0.1 ng/mL at three months, compared with 8.9 ng/mL prior to therapy. While these studies document significant destruction of prostatic tissue, many of the patients were also treated with adjuvant hormonal therapy. Consequently, the significance of the negative biopsies and low PSAs are not obvious and may be of questionable value in assessing outcome. However, the study does document that modern cryotherapy procedures can be completed safely, with the major side effects being incontinence (3%), rare stricture, sloughing of urethral tissue, and urinary retention (41). No patients developed rectourethral or urethrocutaneous fistulas (41).

Cryosurgical ablation has also been used in an attempt to salvage patients who have failed locally following radiation therapy, androgen ablation, or both (40). In preliminary data reported from the University of Texas M. D. Anderson Cancer Center, 76 patients in whom radiation therapy failed and who had biopsy-proven locally recurrent disease were treated with cryotherapy (36). In this series with relatively short follow-up, many patients showed a decline in PSA (97%) which was undetectable (<0.1 ng/mL) in 28%. However, complication rates were much greater in this group than in the previously reported study of cryotherapy as primary intervention (41). Only 14% of patients escaped complications. Incontinence was present at six months in 31%, impotence occurred in 49%, pain in 25%, urinary obstruction in 24%, and severe hematuria in 13%. Additional studies with longer follow-up will be necessary to define the efficacy and complication rates in men treated with cryotherapy after radiotherapy.

■ CONCLUSION

Theoretically, cryotherapy has the potential to become one of the useful therapies for prostate cancer in selected individuals. However, physicians and patients must realize that long-term results are not available with regard to efficacy and complications. Cryotherapy should be offered to patients only as part of a controlled study, so that objective data can be obtained.

Editorial Comment

Brachytherapy (the implantation of radioactive seeds) and cryotherapy are old technologies that have been resurrected in the modern era primarily because of the availability of better imaging techniques. In regard to brachytherapy, the authors provide an important historical perspective, namely that the "freehand" placement of radioactive seeds was inferior to both external beam radiation and surgery in terms of local control. This led many large centers to abandon brachytherapy as a treatment option for localized prostate cancer 15 to 20 years ago.

The modern series using transrectal ultrasound- or CT-guided seed placement is encouraging. However, enthusiasm must be tempered by the fact that long-term follow-up (10 years later) for brachytherapy using modern imaging is nonexistent. A similar shortcoming, in terms of length of follow-up and number of patients reported, exists regarding potency data and local complication rates.

Cryosurgery, like brachytherapy, is old technology that has been reexamined in the modern era because of the improvement in imaging techniques. Again, there is no long-term follow-up available for any of the modern series. The preliminary experience does report what appears to be a very high rate of complications, including incontinence, impotence, pain, urinary obstruction, and severe hematuria.

Brachytherapy and cryosurgery represent old therapeutic modalities that are now being reapplied to the treatment of localized prostate cancer. Clinicians who treat prostate cancer realize that it is treacherous to draw conclusions regarding this disease based on small cohorts of patients or short-term follow-up. These caveats should be remembered as we analyze the current experience with these two treatment modalities.

■ REFERENCES

1. Wallner K, Roy J, Zelefsky M, et al. Fluoroscopic visualization of the prostatic urethra to guide transperineal prostate implantation. Int J Radiat Oncol Biol Phys 1994;29:863–867.
2. Holm HH, et al. Transperineal ^{125}iodine seed implantation in prostate cancer guided by transrectal ultrasound. J Urol 1983;103:283–287.

3. Wallner K, Chiu-Tsao S, Roy J, et al. A new device to stabilize templates for transperineal I-125 implants. Int J Radiat Oncol Biol Phys 1991;20:1075–1077.

4. Scardino PT, Carlton CE. Combined interstitial and external irradiation for prostatic cancer. In: Jevadpour N, ed. Principles and management of urologic cancer. Baltimore: Williams and Wilkins, 1983:392–408.

5. Whitmore WF. Interstitial I-125 implantation in the management of prostate cancer. Prog Clin Biol Res 1984;153:513–527.

6. Koprowski CD, Berkenstock KG, Borofski AM, et al. External beam irradiation versus 125 iodine implant in the definitive treatment of prostate carcinoma. Int J Radiat Oncol Biol Phys 1991;21:955–960.

7. Kuban DA, Anas EM, Schellhammer PF. I-125 interstitial implantation for prostate cancer: what have we learned 10 years later? Cancer 1989;63:2415–2420.

8. Morton JD, Peschel RE. Iodine-125 implants versus external beam therapy for stages A2, B, and C prostate cancer. Int J Radiat Oncol Biol Phys 1988;14:1153–1157.

9. Priestly JB. Use of MICK applicator in transperineal ultrasound-guided ^{125}I seed implantation. J Endourol 1990;4:375–379.

10. Kaye KW, Olson DJ, Lightner DJ, et al. Improved technique for prostate seed-implantation: combined ultrasound and fluoroscopic guidance. J Endourol 1992;6:61–66.

11. Wallner K, Roy J, Zelefsky M, et al. Short-term freedom from disease progression after I-125 prostate implantation. Int J Radiat Oncol Biol Phys 1994;30:405–409.

12. Priestly JB, Beyer DC. Guided brachytherapy for treatment of confined prostate cancer. Urology 1992;40:27–32.

13. Russo SA, Whittington R, Broderick GA, et al. American Urological Association Abstract, 1995.

14. Blasko JC, Grimm PD, Ragde H. Brachytherapy and organ preservation in the management of carcinoma of the prostate. Semin Radiat Oncol 1993;3:240–249.

15. Catalona WJ, Smith DS. Five-year tumor recurrence rates after anatomical radical retropubic prostatectomy for prostate cancer. J Urol 1994;152:1837–1842.

16. Walsh PC, Partin AW, Epstein JI. Cancer control and quality of life following anatomical radical retropubic prostatectomy: results at 10 years. J Urol 1994;152:1831–1836.

17. Bagshaw MA, Cox RS, Hancock SL. Control of prostate cancer with radiotherapy: long-term results. J Urol 1994;152:1781–1785.

18. Bagshaw MA, Ray GR, Cox RA. Complications associated with radiotherapy of prostate cancer. In: Smith RB, Ehrlich RM, eds. Complications of urologic surgery: prevention and management. 2nd ed. Philadelphia: WB Saunders, 1990:88–99.

19. Talcott JA, Rieker P, Propert K, et al. Complications of treatment for early prostate cancer: a prospective, multi-institutional outcome study. Proc Annu Meet Am Soc Clin Oncol 1994;13:A711. Abstract.

20. Hanks GE, Hanlon A, Schultheiss T, et al. Early prostate cancer: national results of radiation treatment from patterns of care and radiation therapy oncology group studies with prospects for improvement with conformal radiation and adjuvant androgen deprivation. J Urol 1994;152:1775–1780.

21. Liebel SA, Zelefsky MJ, Kutcher GJ, et al. Three-dimensional conformal radiation therapy in localized carcinoma of the prostate: interim report of phase I dose escalation study. J Urol 1994;152:1792–1798.

22. Shipley WU, Zietman AL, Hanks GE, et al. Treatment related sequelae following external beam radiation therapy for prostate cancer: review with update in patients with stages T1 and T2 tumor. J Urol 1994;152:1799–1805.

23. Zietman AL, Coen JJ, Shipley WU, et al. Radical radiation therapy in the management of prostatic adenocarcinoma: the initial prostate specific antigen value as a predictor of treatment outcome. J Urol 1994;151:640–645.

24. Zagars GK. Prostate specific antigen as an outcome variable for T1 and T2 prostate cancer treated by radiation therapy. J Urol 1994;152:1786–1791.

25. Rosen MA, Goldstone L, Lapin S, et al. Frequency and location of extracapsular extension and positive surgical margins in radical prostatectomy specimens. J Urol 1992;148:331–337.

26. Epstein JI, Pizov G, Walsh PC. Correlation of pathologic findings with progression after radical retropubic prostatectomy. Cancer 1993;71:3582–3593.

27. D'Amico AV, Whittington R, Malkowicz SB, et al. A multivariable analysis of clinical factors predicting for pathological features associated with local failure after radical prostatectomy for prostate cancer. Int J Radiat Oncol Biol Phys 1994;30:293–302.

28. Oesterling JE, Suman VJ, Zincke H, et al. PSA-detected (clinical stage T1c or B0) prostate cancer. Urol Clin North Am 1993;20:687–693.

29. Epstein JI, Walsh PC, Carmichael M, et al. Pathologic and clinical

findings to predict tumor extent of nonpalpable (stage T1c) prostate cancer. JAMA 1994;271:368–374.

30. Partin AW, Yoo J, Carter HB, et al. The use of prostate specific antigen, clinical stage and Gleason score to predict pathological stage in men with localized prostate cancer. J Urol 1993;150:110–114.

31. Catalona WJ, Dresner SM. Nerve-sparing radical prostatectomy: extraprostatic tumor extension and preservation of erectile function. J Urol 1985;134:1149–1153.

32. Littrup PJ, Montie J, Ashish M, et al. Prostatic cryotherapy: ultrasonographic and pathologic correlation in the canine model. Urology 1994;44:175–184.

33. Gonder MJ, Soanes WA, Smith V. Experimental prostate cryosurgery. Invest Urol 1964;1:610.

34. Gonder MJ, Soanes WA, Shulman S. Cryosurgical treatment of the prostate. Invest Urol 1966;3:372.

35. Flocks RH, Nelson CMK, Boatman DL. Perineal cryosurgery for prostate carcinoma. J Urol 1972;108:933–935.

36. Bonney WW, Fallon B, Gerber WL, et al. Cryosurgery in prostate cancer: survival. Urology 1982;19:37–42.

37. Onik GM, Cobb C, Cohen J, et al. US characteristics of frozen prostate. Radiology 1988;168:629–631.

38. Onik GM, Porterfield B, Rubinsky B, et al. Percutaneous prostate cryosurgery using transrectal ultrasound guidance: animal model. Urology 1991;72:1291–1299.

39. Onik GM, Cohen J, Reyes GD, et al. Transrectal ultrasound-guided ablation of the prostate. Cancer 1993;72:1291–1299.

40. Dinney PN, Pisters LL, Von Eschenbach AC. Cryoablation for prostate cancer. In: Vogelzang, et al., eds. Comprehensive textbook of genitourinary oncology. Baltimore: Williams and Wilkins, 1996:828–837.

41. Miller RJ, Cohen JK, Merlotti LA. Percutaneous transperineal cryosurgical ablation of the prostate for the primary treatment of clinical stage C adenocarcinoma of the prostate. Urology 1994;44:170–184.

Patient Treatment Choices and Outcomes in Early Prostate Cancer

9

▼ ▼ ▼ ▼ ▼ ▼ ▼ ▼

James A. Talcott
Clair J. Beard
Kenneth I. Wishnow

F OR MOST potentially curable cancers, which may progress from diagnosis to death within a year, patients' treatment options are few, their role in decision making is limited, and their treatment goal is survival, primarily if not solely. The rationale for toxic therapies—that prolonged life outweighs almost any short-term unpleasantness and danger—is valid, and discussion of quality of life is moot.

Declaring a personal, no-holds-barred war on cancer may be more attractive to patients now than ever, because cancer and cancer therapy have gone public, making the ordeal of cancer treatment less secretive and private. Heads recently denuded of hair by chemotherapy, once covered by medically prescribed wigs, gleam in public more often, shown in bittersweet defiance as badges of courage. Some fight the War on Cancer, declared by President Nixon nearly a quarter century ago, with fresh fury, as in women's headlined legal battles for access to bone marrow transplants for breast cancer and the public campaigns for more research dollars. Bright publicity greets newly announced treatments, such as interferon or adaptive immunotherapy with lymphokine-activated killer (LAK) cells, although this seeps slowly away as less publicized studies disprove early, optimistic claims.

This aggressive approach provides the context for most people seeking treatment for newly diagnosed cancer. However, the fights against these aggressive cancers echo only faintly and perhaps confusingly for men with early (nonmetastatic) prostate cancer. The difference is not that prostate cancer is an unimportant malady. It is a potentially lethal neoplasm, killing tens of thousands annually in brief, relentless progressions of painful bone metastases and hypermetabolic inanition. However, prostate cancer doesn't kill the great majority of patients in whom it is found, and often when death comes, years have passed since diagnosis. For most of its long natural history, prostate cancer progresses silently and without symptoms, during the later years of men's lives, when other potentially fatal illnesses may emerge and independently erode health. Other than by obstructing urine flow, prostate cancer can be expected to have little effect on most men's health for years after diagnosis.

Like most cancers, prostate cancer does not kill until and unless it becomes metastatic. For this usually slow-growing cancer, the progression from confinement within the prostate capsule to symptomatic metastatic disease often takes a decade or more. The goal of potentially curative local therapy, such as radical prostatectomy of external beam radiotherapy, is to eradicate all cancer completely before metastatic seeds of destruction spread to the bones. When it becomes metastatic, it is incurable. If cancer has escaped the prostate before treatment, the effort to cure will be entirely in vain, although years will probably pass before the failure becomes evident. Thus, treatment is separated from its intended effect, the prevention of metastatic cancer, by a span of years, the time it takes for localized disease to progress to clinically evident metastases. Treating prostate cancer may prevent a terrible outcome, but much time must pass for its result to be felt, if ever.

Other than its comparatively slow rate of natural progression, the most important characteristic of prostate cancer to be kept in mind when choosing treatment is that it occurs in older men. It is rare before age 50 but rises in frequency, becoming extraordinarily common, as men grow old. Microscopic prostate cancer is found in the prostates of more men than not who die of other causes after age 70, and it can be found in nearly 80% of men in their eighties. While the clinical diagnosis of prostate cancer is much less common, it too rises steeply with age. Of the approximately 11% of men found to have it during their lifetime, more than half are diagnosed after age 70. However, the explosive spread of screening using the prostate-specific antigen (PSA) doubled the rate at which prostate cancer was diagnosed between 1991 and 1995, enabling the diagnosis of cancers earlier and lowering the average age at diagnosis. While diagnosing so many early cancers has raised hopes that deaths from prostate cancer will fall, definitive results are not in. Unfortunately, simply diagnosing cancer at an earlier age does not necessarily make death from cancer come later. To benefit men, earlier diagnosis must make treatment more effective. Otherwise, the portion of life a man lives with known cancer simply expands at the expense of the period before.

Because men who have localized prostate cancer generally live many years with the disease, and most are diagnosed when older, they and their peers are likely to encounter other potentially debilitating and lethal diseases. Health goals often change as one progresses from one's forties to one's sixties, seventies, and eighties. Avoiding death by prostate cancer yields a smaller bonus of additional life than can be won from other cancers, which strike earlier and progress more rapidly. A man with prostate cancer diagnosed in his late sixties and early seventies has usually seen death among friends, family members, and acquaintances of his age, and has begun to think of death as an unavoidable factor in his coming years. It has been said in bittersweet jest that the problem with prolonging life is that the extra years come when one is old. Life is a treasure, but for most people, waning natural powers and accumulating bodily afflictions color the experience of advancing years. For most young persons, the value of trading unpleasant cancer therapy for additional years of life is obvious and not usually questioned. However, for men in their sixties and seventies, the value of exchanging a chance for additional years in ones' eighties for a possible additional physical burden is more ambiguous. Thus, for many men with prostate cancer, the end of their life is foreseeable, and the trade-off of quality of life for prolonged life is understood to be a compact with an expiration date.

For prostate cancer treatment, the trade-off of diminished quality of life for an attempt to prolong it may not be limited to the period of active treatment and immediately thereafter: the bowel, bladder, and sexual dysfunction after treatment for prostate cancer may be prolonged or permanent. Most men have sexual dysfunction or urinary incontinence for several months after radical prostatectomy, with recovery usually extending through the first year. And while some men who are still incontinent or impotent a year after radical prostatectomy may still regain continence or potency, most will not. Further, men who retain sexual potency a year after radiotherapy for prostate cancer may still lose it during the next. Thus, the disabilities following treatment of prostate cancer may not only not resolve, but may also even progress in some cases.

The prolonged recovery period during which lost sexual and urinary function after radical prostatectomy or radical radiotherapy may improve or further erode may leave men feeling uncertain for months or even years. Waiting uncertainly for recovery can give men time to adapt to their changed circumstances and get on with their lives, but it can also distract them from acceptance and adaptation.

For most men, any major functional impairment present a year after therapy is unlikely to improve spontaneously, although some conditions may benefit from treatment. These impairments represent long-term dysfunction, the price paid in advance to defend against a dreaded cancer's return years hence. This trade-off does not precisely represent delayed gratification. Instead, the gratification of sexual function or effortless and well-controlled bowel or bladder function may be postponed permanently. Thus, the fundamental bargain into which a prostate cancer patient must enter is to place at risk one's usual level of function in one or more areas of intimate bodily function in exchange for possibly postponing death and avoiding the pain of death from cancer.

Although all the treatments for prostate cancer may affect bowel, urinary, and sexual function, the array of potential difficulties varies from treatment to treatment. For example, radical prostatectomy entails a substantial risk of urinary incontinence, while external beam radiotherapy often causes bowel and bladder irritation. Further, the time course is different for surgery and radiotherapy complications. Radical prostatectomy patients have their worst sexual and urinary dysfunction immediately after the operation, with only improvements expected in the year or two ahead. With external beam radiation, things flow less directly. For a few weeks before and after the radiotherapy course is completed, a subacute period of irritative symptoms of bowel and bladder may occur, many of which resolve within the first year. However, the gradual process of scar formation after radiation may result in gradually weakened erections, as the nerves that steer blood flow to the penis during arousal become damaged and the valves that hold the blood within the penis accumulate leakage. While the time course of dysfunction is for most men not as important as its probability and severity, understanding the process may help many men adapt to it. Therefore, men need to know both what can be expected to happen to them and when.

The information available to most men about the complications they can expect after prostate cancer treatment has likely been unreliable, underestimating their chances of having problems. The fundamental difficulty is the virtual absence of the unbiased data, the best of which come from randomized clinical trials. In these trials, which are the "gold standard" design for clinical research, eligible patients are assigned their treatment by chance, rather receiving the researcher's preferred therapy. Because chance alone determines the treatment received, patients go into treatment, on average, with an equal chance of dying of cancer or of another cause. Similarly, they have an equal chance of experiencing complications of treatment. Therefore, any difference found in the overall outcomes of the patient groups is due to the treatments themselves, rather than to some other confounding variable causing patients with the best prognoses to be steered to one or the other treatment. Despite the value of randomized trials, prominent authorities commonly state that a large randomized trial of prostate cancer therapy is impossible to complete, because patients and doctors have strong treatment preferences (1). Even if they didn't, the argument goes on, the treatments are so different from one another (and from observation alone) that having one's choice determined by chance just doesn't sit well with patients. However, to an outsider the problem appears ideal to study, since it is so important, so many patients have the diagnosis, and we know so little with certainty about its treatment. With at least 150,000 men diagnosed annually with prostate cancer without clinical evidence of tumor spread, and with a generally acknowledged uncertainty about which treatments are better, or even of value, one might expect to find abundant doctor and patient enthusiasm for such a trial. In any case, such trials have not been completed. In the absence of results from such randomized trials, patients and doctors are forced to rely on lesser sources of information. Unfortunately, these have, until recently, been much less reliable.

The most common sources of information about treatment complications are data from what are known as treatment case series. In these studies, an individual physician or a group of physicians who treat prostate cancer patients, usually specializing in only one treatment, such as prostatectomy or radiation therapy, keeps track of the patients treated and publishes the outcomes. The advantage of this sort of report is that it allows patients and doctors access to the experience of large numbers of patients treated in one way. An interested reader can then contrast the results of patients treated with one treatment with the results of treatment alternatives. Until recently, just these sorts of comparisons have dominated the study of treatment-related quality of life (as well as the efficacy of treatment). Unfortunately, such comparisons may be seriously misleading, largely like comparing apples to oranges (2). The basic analytical problem is that patients may be selected for a particular treatment because they have characteristics that influence how well they will do, quite apart from the effects of treatment. If that is true, the patients have different prognoses even before treatment, making it nearly impossible to determine what effect the treatment itself had on their outcome. This situation certainly pertains to prostate cancer. Since diagnosing prostate cancer requires a biopsy, a surgical procedure, the first doctor offering treatment advice to most prostate cancer patients is a urologist. Most surgeons feel radical prostatectomy is the preferred treatment for most patients (just as most radiotherapists prefer radiotherapy) (1). However, some patient characteristics tend to make urologists discourage or refuse surgery and recommend radiation therapy or even observation instead. Among these factors are older age (with upper age limits usually at 65 to 75 years); serious enough heart, lung, or other medical problems to make surviving a two- to three-hour-long radical prostatectomy operation risky; and evidence of cancer spread through the prostate capsule, making it unlikely that it will be completely removed by surgery. While such selection criteria are sensible and thoughtful, they result in the surgery patient group's being systematically different from that of radiotherapy patients. Surgery patients as a group are younger, healthier, and have less advanced cancers, while radiotherapy patients are older and are more likely to have both serious noncancer "comorbid" conditions and larger, more advanced cancers. As a result, surgery patients have brighter futures than radiation therapy patients, regardless of the effects of treatment, and this hopelessly confuses comparisons of the patient groups' outcomes after treatment. Making matters worse, most reports of case series don't include the most important patient prognostic information, such as the Gleason score, patient age, and extent of comorbid diseases (3).

This problem of unequal comparisons may be easier to understand for comparisons of treatment based on survival than on such outcomes as impotence or radiation proctitis. Given this so-called selection bias, it is easier to see why surgery patients are likely to live longer than radiation therapy patients than it is to see why the older, sicker radiation therapy patients are more likely to have incontinence or problems with erections before their treatment or to develop them afterward. However, knowing the status of a patient's bowel, bladder, and sexual functioning before treatment makes the comparison between treatment groups more informative. Without knowing the patient's prior status, the relative contributions of treatment and pretreatment status to complications will always be unclear.

Another important problem with the evidence from case series arises because the doctors who treat the cancer are usually same ones who ask patients if they have developed treatment-related complications. The close, interdependent relationship between doctor and patient may inhibit communication. Cancer patients are both grateful for and dependent on their doctors' efforts on their behalf and may be reluctant to complain. To some patients, reporting problems makes them "bad patients." It is a common experience for doctors to hear from a family member or a nurse of a complaint that, when asked directly, the patient denies or minimizes. This phenomenon may importantly reduce the complications reported. Further, doctors may subconsciously signal their own lack of enthusiasm for hearing about complications. The doctor who publishes his or her patients' results is putting his or her professional expertise on display. In general, most persons are relatively more alert to positive than negative feedback. Without making careful, conscious efforts to ask clear, understandable questions to clarify patients' vague or ambiguous responses, physicians may inadvertently diminish the complications they record and report.

To avoid some of these data collection problems in patient treatment series, some more recent studies have avoided having the treating physicians ask the questions (4–6). Instead, third parties not involved with treatment conduct the patient interviews or questionnaires. In addition, survey research techniques are used to craft unambiguous, easily understood questions that have clearly defined and comprehensive answers. Not surprisingly, given the known problems with earlier studies, these recent studies found substantially higher complication rates. The contrast between results obtained in this more objective way and the previously published case series can be striking at times. For example, very large series by two of the best-know urologic surgery groups in the United States reported overall incontinence rates of less than 10% (7,8). However, two retrospective direct surveys of patients (4,5) and our own prospective survey (6) found incontinence rates of 40% to 73%. Similarly, impotence rates following radical prostatectomy were reported by the same investigators as being between 25% and 50%, but according to the direct patient surveys, impotence rates range from 52% to 93%, depending in part on the definition of potency. While other factors, including the definition of the complication, may account for some variation in results, differences of this magnitude are probably due to the difference in the data collection technique. We believe that the most valid results come when third parties survey patients directly, using well-tested, unambiguous questions. When these more objective techniques are used, higher complication rates are found. Therefore, in this chapter we give substantially greater weight to the latter, direct patient surveys than the earlier case series.

■ BASIC TREATMENT CHOICES AND THEIR COMPLICATIONS

Radical Prostatectomy

The most common treatment choice for patients with early prostate cancer today is radical prostatectomy, which has increased dramatically over the past decade (9). This surgical technique completely excises the prostate, the prostatic urethra, and the seminal vesicles. The complications of radical prostatectomy primarily fall into four categories: 1) those resulting from the operative procedure itself and general anesthesia, including intraoperative and perioperative complications; 2) loss of sexual erections; 3) urinary incontinence; and 4) postsurgical scarring, or strictures, which obstruct urine flow. Each of these deserves a brief discussion.

The risk of operative and postoperative death appears to be falling. While death rates in some series in the late 1970s were as high as 3% to 4% (3), most contemporary series from major centers report death rates well under the commonly cited figure of 1% (10). Several factors may contribute to this, including better surgical and anesthesia techniques in the operating room, improved detection and treatment of complications after surgery, and a healthier group of patients being operated on, because younger patients are being detected by screening and there is more careful selection now to exclude the older, sicker patients at higher risk. The primary danger to patients during general anesthesia is a heart attack, an irregular heart rhythm, or a stroke. In the period after the operation, blood clots in the legs (deep venous thrombosis) may occur and, at worst, break off and go to the lungs (pulmonary embolus). One or more of these complications occurs in 2% to 3% of patients who undergo radical prostatectomy.

Sexual impotence was, until 10 or 15 years ago, presumed after radical prostatectomy, a side effect that certainly contributed to its relative unpopularity. However, Walsh and colleagues at Johns Hopkins University performed anatomic studies that documented the importance of two neurovascular bundles running along either side of the prostate. When Walsh identified and left these structures intact in the reversed operation he devised, the so-called nerve-sparing radical prostatectomy, a surprising number of patients had erections adequate for sexual intercourse after the procedure (11,12). Potency is not continuous through surgery and its aftermath. Almost all men lose erections immediately after radical prostatectomy; the trauma of the procedure appears to be too much for the rather delicate and complex human erection. However, as time passes, many men regain their ability to have erections. Walsh has reported that most patients report the return of sexual function after the nerve-sparing, or (as he now prefers to call it) "anatomic," radical prostatectomy. In fact, Walsh reported that as many as three-fourths of young men (under age 60) with small or nonpalpable tumors were able to have intercourse after radical prostatectomy (13). Other surgeons have been unable to quite replicate such good results, but most report the preservation of full sexual functioning in many men after this procedure. One factor in the difference between Walsh's data and those of others may simply be surgical skill; Walsh developed the retropubic nerve-sparing operation, is certainly its best-known practitioner, and has performed it hundreds of times. However, his patients are also highly selected for favorable preoperative characteristics. Because of his national reputation, many men come to him to be evaluated for prostate surgery, and only the best candidates among them are chosen. Thus, Walsh's patients tend to be young and to have small tumors, compared with patients operated on by other surgeons, even at his own Johns Hopkins Medical School. Other investigators whose patients are older and have larger tumors, such as Catalona of Washington University, report impotence in half of patients or more (8). In addition, Walsh has obtained his complication rates by asking patients directly about their erections, a setting in which patients may not be completely forthcoming. The results of more recent direct patient surveys show the higher impotence rates we mentioned earlier, with complete impotence rates of 52% to 78%.

It should be remembered that a treatment plan may change after it gets under way because of new information. Therefore, the treatment a patient chose may not be exactly what he gets, particularly in the case of nerve-sparing radical prostatectomy. The nerve-sparing procedure requires a surgeon to cut around a delicate structure, the neurovascular bundle, which is adjacent to the capsule of the prostate. Ensuring that the bundle is preserved runs the risk of leaving at least microscopic fragments of prostate behind. While there is no harm in leaving healthy prostate behind, prostate cancer tends to be multifocal (existing in several places within the prostate), so that leaving prostate *tissue* behind entails a risk of leaving prostate *cancer* behind. Therefore, a surgeon must make the decision during the operation that no cancer appears to be too near either neurovascular bundle he is attempting to preserve. A surgeon who fully intends to perform a bilateral nerve-sparing prostatectomy may find at surgery that the tumor approaches both bundles too closely for comfort, and instead perform a non-nerve-sparing prostatectomy. More often, the tumor approaches only one bundle, and the surgeon then attempts nerve preservation on only one side. This means that some patients who choose nerve-sparing prostatectomy will not get it at all, and that others will receive only unilateral nerve sparing. While more objective studies have not been able to measure the relative potency benefits of the unilateral and bilateral versions of the nerve-sparing technique, some recent reports, including the preliminary results from our own study, show that if only one neurovascular bundle is spared, the benefits are minimal (14,14a). The best published potency rates after nerve-sparing prostatectomy are reported for men who underwent bilateral nerve-sparing prostatectomy, which is a subset of surgery patients with the best results. It is important for patients to understand that not all of those who choose the bilateral nerve-sparing procedure will be lucky enough to get it, and that the results for patients who do are better than average.

In a few cases, other information from tests performed to evaluate the extent of cancer (staging), administer treatment, or perform routine surveillance after treatment results in different or additional treatment. For example, radical prostatectomy is usually preceded by lymph node "sampling," or surgical removal of lymph nodes. If cancer is found in the lymph nodes, eventual metastatic cancer is assumed to be a near certainty, making it futile to proceed to radical prostatectomy, since a local treatment directed solely at cancer still in the pelvis has no effect on metastatic cancer, which alone causes death from prostate cancer. Therefore, when cancer is found in the lymph nodes, the surgeon aborts the planned radical prostatectomy. Then, in lieu of further surgery, the patient is offered hormone ablation therapy (removal of the testes or shots that accomplish the same effect) or initial observation. In a similar vein, if after radical prostatectomy the pathologist finds cancer present at the surgical margin, the cut edge of the prostate tissue, the chance that cancer was left behind is substantial, and additional adjuvant radiotherapy may be recommended. Such changes are unplanned but foreseeable possible consequences of choosing radical prostatectomy. These changes of plan are important, since patient results are usually presented according to the treatment patients actually received rather than the treatment they initially chose. Such results are potentially misleading, since some patients who chose a particular therapy are excluded from the results—often those expected to fare the worst. A series may report the results of only those who had radical prostatectomy alone, excluding patients who received adjuvant radiotherapy or hormonal therapy. The excluded patients requiring additional treatments have the larger, more aggressive tumors, which more often cannot be completely resected or have spread to lymph nodes. Thus the reported outcomes may be significantly better than for all patients who chose radical prostatectomy, artificially lowering complication rates. Patients must therefore be careful about applying published results to themselves.

The third major complication of radical prostatectomy is urinary incontinence. This occurs because the prostate lies very close to the muscles that clench and relax, preventing urine from leaking out of the bladder or letting it flow, as the patient desires. Some postoperative incontinence in some men seems to be impossible to avoid. For many men, the leakage occurs at only certain times and under certain conditions. For example, in the act of standing up, the abdominal muscles involuntarily contract, making the body more rigid and the muscles more effective in raising it to the standing position. This raises the pressure inside the abdomen, pressing down on the bladder and forcing the sphincter to work harder to prevent urine from leaking out. Urine leakage at times like this is called stress incontinence, and it occurs at other times as well, including when the patient coughs or makes other sudden movements. While urinary incontinence rates are usually reported at less than 10%, more recent surveys directly canvassing patients found that 30% to 40% of men are incontinent at least sometimes, and that about one-third of men wear pads in their underwear to absorb leaked urine. For most men the leakage is a minor annoyance, but for others, perhaps 10%, the incontinence is a bigger problem. For these men, the problem may simply require changing absorptive pads once or twice a day; more severely affected men may require a clamp on the penis.

Finally, urethral strictures arise because the healing process after radical prostatectomy causes scars to form. These fibrous bands may obstruct the flow of urine if they happen to stretch across the urethral channel. If these strictures do cause urinary obstruction, they can be stretched out by a urologist while the urethra itself has been numbed with a local anesthetic.

In summary, a patient choosing radical prostatectomy will undergo a major surgical procedure that uncommonly results in a heart attack, stroke, blood clots, and even death. Probably he will become sexually impotent. The risk of impotence is lessened if he undergoes the nerve-sparing procedure, but whether he will actually receive it depends in part on what the surgeon discovers at surgery. Urinary incontinence is at least an occasional problem for one-third of men, although only about 10% leak a lot. Finally, some men develop obstruction to urinary flow from a urethral stricture, a problem that can be repaired with a minor urologic procedure.

■ RADIOTHERAPY

Although radical prostatectomy is the most common choice for men with early prostate cancer, thousands of men annually choose to undergo radiation therapy for prostate cancer. Their reasons vary. Some who were refused prostatectomy because of locally advanced disease (cancer spread through the prostate capsule) choose radiotherapy as the only available "potentially curative" therapy, despite knowing that they are at high risk for already having undetected microscopic metastatic disease, which would make cure impossible. Some early-stage patients with far less advanced disease and the option of surgery choose radiation to avoid the inconvenience of a hospital stay and the prolonged postoperative recovery period, or simply from fear of the prospect of major abdominal surgery and general anesthesia. Older patients and those with significant heart or lung disease may be at higher risk from surgery, and may conclude themselves, or be gently persuaded, that radiation is an easier alternative to get through. Others may be persuaded by the much lower risk of incontinence or the later onset and possibly lower incidence of impotence compared with radical prostatectomy (and accept the greater chance of bowel problems). These patients are choosing what they feel is the "less morbid" treatment, despite the possibility that radiation may be less efficacious than radical prostatectomy, implying a willingness to trade quantity for quality of life. Each option makes sense to some patients, while other patients with the same information may consider it a poor choice.

As men with prostate cancer sift through the assumptions, biases, and the shaky evidence available in an effort to make their treatment choice, they realize they need accurate information about the morbidity of the treatments they are considering and how they might affect the quality of their life. As for radical prostatectomy, few prospective data are available regarding radiation-related morbidity, and some existing data call others into question. One prospective study of radiation therapy patients undergoing external beam irradiation found that medical staff consistently underestimated treatment-related toxicity, compared with patient reports (15). With these issues in mind, we review radiation-induced morbidity and the technical and patient-related factors that contribute to it.

Most patients who choose irradiation receive standard external beam treatment. High-energy x-ray beams (photons) are directed at the prostate, seminal vesicles, and proximal urethra via a four-field approach, through the front, back, and sides of the patient. Some clinicians also treat pelvic lymph nodes, to sterilize any micrometastases within them. Treating lymph nodes is controversial, because little evidence exists supporting the belief that irradiating cancerous lymph nodes will prolong life, probably because cancer in lymph nodes signals the likely presence of other metastatic cancer elsewhere. A course of typical radiation therapy consists of daily treatment, five times per week, for approximately eight weeks. The goal of planning treatment fields is to consistently expose the target (prostate) to the radiation beam while minimizing irradiation of the surrounding normal tissues. For prostate cancer patients, the important nearby normal tissues are the bladder, the rectum, and the neurovascular bundles. The last, the structures implicated in developing erections, lie within the periprostatic fat. Radiation works by damaging the DNA and other crucial molecules within exposed cells, both directly and by generating highly reactive oxygen fragments. Affected cells die either when they attempt to divide or when the preprogrammed process of dying (apoptosis) is triggered by other damage. Normal tissue can as a rule better repair radiation damage than neoplastic tissue, which thus succumbs more easily to radiation treatment. Side effects occur during and after irradiation and can be both direct, from direct radiation damage to normal tissue, and indirect, as a result of the body's attempts to repair radiation changes (inflammation and scarring). The most common side effects are: 1) fatigue, 2) gastrointestinal dysfunction, 3) bladder irritation, and 4) sexual dysfunction. In general, irritative gastrointestinal and genitourinary side effects are frequent during irradiation but improve substantially by 12 months after treatment, as healing progresses in the normal tissues of the bladder and rectum. However, problems with erections continue to increase for two or more years after irradiation, because of progressive scarring of the nerves and perhaps related damage to the valves that keep blood in the engorged penis.

Intuitively, a relationship between the type and extent of radiation technique and treatment-related morbidity is plausible. Based on the conclusion of a large, multi-institutional, retrospective review of national radiotherapy practices, that doses of at least 65 grays (Gy) were needed to "sterilize" prostate cancer (16), most radiation oncologists deliver doses between 65 and 70 Gy to prostate cancer patients. A higher dose may be given in experimental dose-escalation protocols, but only with special precautions to shield normal tissue. Within the usual range of 65 to 70 Gy, morbidity goes up along with the volume of treated tissue. When patients receive radiation treatment to large areas of their bladder and rectum, in an attempt to treat pelvic lymph nodes or large seminal vesicles, for example, one can expect greater side effects than when treatment fields are small, directed at the prostate alone. The radiation oncologist chooses large or small fields based on his or her personal preferences, the patient's stage of disease, and the presence of an enlarged prostate gland or seminal vesicles.

In addition to the technical factors, patient-related factors may also contribute to radiation morbidity. Men who have had prior pelvic radiation cannot undergo radiation again. Although there is no absolute chronologic age beyond which a patient may not be treated, practical issues, such as transportation to and from the radiation facility, must be considered before recommending a course of

outpatient treatment lasting seven to eight weeks. Many clinicians refuse to treat patients with a history of ulcerative colitis, fearing that the colitis-related inflammation and scar tissue will increase bowel complications. Any factor that affects blood vessels, such as high blood pressure, atherosclerosis, diabetes, smoking, or prior pelvic surgery, increases an individual patient's risk of complications for any radiation technique. Also, additional comorbid diseases serious enough to shorten their life expectancy may make men hesitate before initiating any treatment for their prostate cancer, including irradiation.

One of the most common side effects experienced by patients undergoing external beam irradiation is fatigue. What causes this is unknown, and no published reports define how often it occurs or how severely. However, most patients describe decreased energy starting several weeks after treatment begins. It usually lasts for several months after therapy but eventually resolves. Although fatigue isn't experienced by everyone, patients contemplating a course of radiation should expect it. They may require additional rest at night or need to curtail some of their more vigorous activities. The fatigue does not progress to complete exhaustion, and many motivated patients with jobs work throughout their course of treatment.

Permanent gastrointestinal disturbance is reported in 5% to 10% of treated men in the retrospective literature studies. Patients, particularly those receiving treatment to large fields that include the pelvic lymph nodes, may expect mild to moderate diarrhea. This generally responds to dietary modifications or over-the-counter antidiarrhea medications. Patients receiving treatment to smaller fields usually do not develop diarrhea but may develop proctitis, with symptoms of increased gassiness, tenesmus (a painful bowel spasm and sense of having to move one's bowels), urgency, and more frequent bowel movements. Occasionally, patients may pass some blood or mucus with their stool. Dietary changes such as avoidance of caffeine, roughage, and spicy foods may help ease these symptoms. Although corticosteroid-containing medications such as mesalamine (Rowasa) suppositories or hydrocortisone acetate and pramoxine hydrochloride (Proctofoam-HC), speed healing, patients usually feel their symptoms don't warrant drug intervention. In general, gastrointestinal symptoms have a peak incidence during the last weeks of irradiation, with substantial recovery over the next several months. Most patients regain normal bowel function, although recovery may take two years or more (Talcott JA, unpublished observations). Perhaps 10% to 20% of patients are left with permanent noticeable rectal symptoms (Beard C, unpublished observations). Rectal bleeding occurs in two different time periods. Late in the course of radiation or within a month or two of completing it, patients may pass some bright red blood secondary to proctitis or hemorrhoidal irritation. In the months and years following therapy, the blood vessels of the anterior rectal wall become thickened and the mucosa atrophies, making small blood vessels more accessible. Microscopic blood may be detected in the stool of up to 50% of treated patients (Beard, unpublished observations), who are otherwise unaware of the blood and without other symptoms. Most physicians prudently perform a sigmoidoscopy or colonoscopy to rule out other causes of gastrointestinal bleeding. A small percentage of patients, fewer than 5%, may have problematic, continuous bleeding requiring intervention (17).

Presumably bladder symptoms occur because of irritation, inflammation, and swelling of the bladder base or prostatic urethra as the tissues are irradiated. Many patients have urinary problems of blocked or slow urine flow even before treatment because of prostatism or obstruction from the bulk of the cancer itself. Radiation can worsen this so-called urinary outlet obstruction during therapy, but by 12 months after treatment urine flow may be better than before therapy (6). Patients with high-grade outlet obstruction prior to irradiation occasionally become completely obstructed during treatment and require placement of a Foley catheter, a tube placed into the bladder through the penis. Patients report increased urinary frequency, incomplete emptying, urgency, and dysuria. Hematuria, or blood in the urine, may be seen within a month or two of the end of treatment and occasionally in the years following treatment. Up to half of patients undergoing treatment will report some irritative bladder symptoms. Medication to anesthetize the bladder, such as phenazopyridine hydrochloride (Pyridium), or to improve urinary obstruction, such as terazosin hydrochloride (Hytrin), may be prescribed. Like radiation-induced gastrointestinal disturbances, these irritative bladder symptoms are generally at most annoying, and improve substantially during the months following radiation. Long-term incontinence occurs in about 5% of patients over 70 years of age (6).

Unlike those associated with surgery, the effects following radiation therapy are not immediate but rather increase with time. Impotence gradually increases for at least the first two years after radiation therapy, producing complete impotence in about a quarter of men and gradually weakened erections in many more (6). Radiation therapy patients, older and more often impotent before treatment than radical prostatectomy patients, have fewer problems at one year after treatment, but gradually catch up by two years, when 80% to 90% of both surgery and radiation therapy patients are unable to have sexual intercourse. Patients often experience dry or uncomfortable ejaculation and may report a decreased libido. Radiation does not appear to decrease testosterone levels but rather probably damages either the small blood vessels of the neurovascular bundles or the network of veins at the base of the penis.

Radiation oncologists are attempting to improve their results by refining their technique. "Conformal" therapy refers to a new treatment planning and delivery technique that uses computer software to integrate CT images of the patient's internal anatomy, obtained in the radiation therapy treatment position, into treatment planning. This allows a three-dimensional view of the target volume, the prostate and seminal vesicles. The additional information on the position of the prostate within the bony pelvis gives clinicians the confidence to use larger than usual blocks to protect normal tissue. (The blocks conform to the shape of the prostate and seminal vesicles, the basis for the term *conformal therapy*.) However, the additional information comes at a cost. In addition to the specialized equipment required, the treatment planning process is more labor intensive and thus more costly than traditional treatment planning. Although this procedure is generally accepted to be more accurate than traditional treatment planning, there is still limited (but growing) evidence that it reduces complications and improves treatment efficacy in favor of conformal therapy (18,19,19a).

In another approach used in several centers, patients with large, bulky prostate cancers are given hormone therapy prior to external beam treatment, to shrink the prostate and seminal vesicles. In two small trials, the smaller posthormone tumors could be treated with smaller radiation fields, reducing exposure to the adjacent normal tissues, the bladder and rectum (19,20). Whether this approach will lead to fewer complications requires further study of larger numbers of patients, with longer follow-up.

■ OTHER TREATMENTS FOR EARLY PROSTATE CANCER

While the vast majority of patients with early prostate cancer receive radical prostatectomy or external beam radiation, three other approaches are chosen by smaller groups of patients. The first of these is simply no initial treatment at all, an approach also known as observation, watchful waiting, or delayed hormonal therapy. This approach has received more interest recently because evidence that radical prostatectomy and external beam radio-therapy cure many patients is indirect and controversial (2), because recent data show a greater than 80% 10-year survival rate for selected patients who are observed (21,22), and because of the complications of the two most common treatments, as discussed above (4–6). Observation certainly avoids the physical complications caused by radical prostatectomy and external beam radiation therapy; an untreated patient cannot have treatment-related complications. However, untreated prostate cancer may grow and obstruct urine flow, and may contribute to sexual impotence either physically, because it grows outside the prostate into critical adjacent structures such as the neurovascular bundles, or psychologically, because knowing that a cancer is growing at the base of his penis generates fear and uncertainty in the patient. However, what keeps most men from choosing observation is that not treating a cancer is simply unthinkable for most Americans—it's a notion akin to giving up. Others may consider it an entirely reasonable option, given their current situation and understanding, but fear that they will regret the decision in the future. While we know that for many if not most men, simply observing their prostate cancer would not shorten their life expectancy, that knowledge may provide little reassurance to a man who is making a crucial decision about a cancer that may kill him in the future. Further, because the PSA test is regularly administered in follow-up visits for prostate cancer, patients who choose not to have treatment can expect to see the PSA value rise, due both to the effects of age on the noncancerous prostate and to continued growth of their cancer. Because the PSA is a well-known index of the growth of prostate cancer, the patient must be regularly confronted with presumptive evidence that his cancer is growing, or choose not to monitor his PSA at all. This is a very difficult choice, encapsulating the difficult psychological dimension of watchful waiting.

Two additional ways of treating prostate cancer have not been well studied at all, particularly for treatment complications. These include radiation implants, sometimes called "seeds" or, more technically, brachytherapy, and cryotherapy, or freezing the prostate. In the first procedure, radioactive pellets, or seeds, are placed into hollow needles that are then inserted into the prostate parallel to one another, under continuous ultrasound monitoring (23). The theoretical appeal of this procedure is that the radioactive material gives high doses of radiation that act over a very short distance. If the rods are placed perfectly, the prostate itself, in theory, receives very high radiation doses while the surrounding tissues receive little if any. This procedure was first developed in the 1970s, but the results were disappointing, at least in part because the technology was not available for placing the seeds accurately. As a result, some areas almost certainly got too little radiation and others got too much, causing both cancer recurrence and damage to the healthy tissue nearby (24). Modern techniques allowing more accurate needle placement have been developed in the past decade, and the technique is being reexamined with fresh interest (25).

The complications of this procedure would be expected to be similar to that of external beam radiotherapy but, ideally, less frequent and severe. In fact, the complication rates have not been carefully studied so far, although our own group has begun to study the patients given brachytherapy by the most experienced group, using the techniques we have applied to surgery and external beam radiation therapy patients. One unusual complication noted in patients receiving brachytherapy is the development of urinary incontinence two or more years after treatment. Further investigation of these patients found calcification in the urethra, leading to the term *super-*

ficial urethral necrosis. Currently efforts are being made to prevent this by reducing the radiation dose to the urethra.

The other alternative technique, cryotherapy, uses a hypercooled probe to freeze prostate tissues, killing both normal and cancerous prostate tissue. The refrigerated probe turns the tissue into ice, which can be easily identified by ultrasound. The complications of this treatment also have not been well studied. Because most practitioners of this technique freeze both neurovascular bundles, one would expect the rate of sexual impotence after treatment to be very high. The rates of urinary incontinence are not known. If the freezing extends outside the prostate, adjoining tissues can be damaged, and the resulting wounds can be difficult to heal. Occasionally this technique results in the formation of abnormal tunnels, or fistulas, between, for example, the rectum and other pelvic tissues, although experienced practitioners report such complications rapidly decrease as the number of patients they have treated rises. Although cryotherapy has been used to treat men with tumor regrowth after radiotherapy treatment, complications of bleeding and poor wound healing have discouraged its use in that context. Further information and perhaps further refinement of the technique will be necessary before we are able to accurately assess its quality-of-life consequences.

■ CONCLUSION

Choosing a treatment for early prostate cancer is difficult for patients and doctors alike. With most cancers, the fundamental question is how to treat the cancer most effectively, nearly without regard for other consequences of treatment. For many of these cancers, the data supporting a particular treatment are reliable and unambiguous. For prostate cancer, however, the situation is much more difficult, and the treatment question itself may be fundamentally different. Prostate cancer grows slowly and kills men late. Because of this, prostate cancer may resemble less an aggressive, quickly lethal cancer than a chronic disease such as diabetes, which sharply reduces the chance of surviving to extreme old age, but poses little short-term health risk. Choosing a treatment approach to prostate cancer may determine how a patient will live in the coming years and even decades. From one perspective, all of the choices facing patients with early prostate cancer, compared with those with other cancers, are good ones: in virtually every case, except for the unusual patient with a very aggressive cancer, the cancer will not seriously threaten their health for at least several years. However, its treatment may cause complications, for many men materially affecting their well-being for years. Understanding what these side effects are and when they might occur is both necessary to making an informed choice of therapy and, we believe, an essential step in adapting to any complications that do arise. We hope this chapter contributes to both.

Editorial Comment

Decisions regarding the need and type of treatment for patients with early prostate cancer require a detailed evaluation of multiple factors, including a patient's life expectancy, the need for and the likelihood of cure, the need for palliation, the impact of therapy on cure and palliation, and the deleterious effects that treatment has on function and quality of life. Unfortunately, although much has been learned in recent years, many of the pieces of this complex puzzle remain uncertain.

We believe that the physician should function as educator and advocate, rather than as the exclusive decision maker, particularly given the complexity and uncertainty that this disease presents. This has been best stated by Sirmon and Kreisberg in their recent article in the *New England Journal of Medicine*, entitled "The Invisible Patient." They stated that "only the physician is capable of knowing all of the benefits and risks of certain procedures, but as a patient advocate he or she must make absolutely certain that the patient, and perhaps the patient's family, have a clear and accurate understanding that allows informed decision making. The physician must be an educator and a counselor, but not the decision maker unless asked by the patient to assume this role."

■ REFERENCES

1. Moore MJ, O'Sullivan B, Tannock IF. How expert physicians would wish to be treated if they had genitourinary cancer. J Clin Oncol 1988;6:1736–1745.
2. Kantoff PW, Talcott JA. The radical prostatectomy series: apples are not oranges. J Clin Oncol 1994;12:2243–2245. Editorial.

3. Wasson JH, Cushman CC, Bruskewitz RC, et al. A structured literature review of treatment for localized prostate cancer. Prostate Disease Patient Outcome Research Team. Arch Fam Med 1993;2:487–493.

4. Fowler F Jr, Barry MJ, Lu-Yao G, et al. Patient-reported complications and follow-up treatment after radical prostatectomy: the national Medicare experience: 1988–1990 (updated June 1993). Urology 1993;42:622–629.

5. Litwin MS, Hays RD, Fink A, et al. Quality-of-life outcomes in men treated for early prostate cancer. JAMA 1995;273:129–135.

6. Talcott JA, Rieker P, Propert K, et al. Complications of treatment for early prostate cancer: a prospective, multi-institutional outcomes study. Proc Annu Meet Am Soc Clin Oncol 1994;13:A711. Abstract.

7. Steiner MS, Morton RA, Walsh PC. Impact of anatomical radical prostatectomy on urinary continence. J Urol 1991;145:512–514.

8. Catalona WJ, Basler JW. Return of erections and urinary continence following nerve sparing radical retropubic prostatectomy. J Urol 1993;150:905–907.

9. Lu-Yao GL, McLerran D, Wasson J, Wennberg JE. An assessment of radical prostatectomy: time trends, geographic variation, and outcomes. The Prostate Patient Outcomes Research Team. JAMA 1993;269:2633–2636.

10. Kramer BS, Brown ML, Prorok PC, et al. Prostate cancer screening: what we know and what we need to know. Ann Intern Med 1993;119:914–923.

11. Walsh PC, Donker PJ. Impotence following radical prostatectomy: insight into etiology and prevention. J Urol 1982;128:492–497.

12. Walsh PC, Lepor H, Eggleston JC. Radical prostatectomy with preservation of sexual function: anatomical and pathological considerations. Prostate 1983;4:473–485.

13. Walsh PC. Radical prostatectomy, preservation of sexual function, cancer control: the controversy. Urol Clin North Am 1987;14:663–673.

14. Geary ES, Dendinger TE, Freiha FS, Stamey TA. Incontinence and vesicle neck strictures following radical retropubic prostatectomy. Urology 1995;45:1000–1006.

14a. Talcott JA, Rieker P, Propert K, et al. Are the potency-sparing benefits of herve-sparing radical prostatectomy due to patient selection? Proc Annu Meet Am Soc Clin Oncol 1995;14:237.

15. Watkins-Bruner D, Scott C, Lawton C, et al. RTOG's first quality of life study, RTOG 900-20: a phase II trial of external beam radiation with

etanidazole for locally advanced prostate cancer. Int J Radiat Oncol Biol Phys 1995.

16. Leibel SA, Hanks GE, Kramer S. Patterns of care outcome studies: results of the national practice in adenocarcinoma of the prostate. Int J Radiat Oncol Biol Phys 1984;10:401–409.

17. Smit WG, Helle PA, Van Putten WL, et al. Late radiation damage in prostate cancer patients treated by high dose external radiotherapy in relation to rectal dose. Int J Radiat Oncol Biol Phys 1990:18:23–29.

18. Hanks GE. Conformal radiation in prostate cancer: reduced morbidity with hope of increased local control. Int J Radiat Oncol Biol Phys 1993;25:377–378. Editorial.

19. Zelefsky MJ, Leibel SA, Burman CM, et al. Neoadjuvant hormonal therapy improves the therapeutic ratio in patients with bulky prostatic cancer treated with three-dimensional conformal radiation therapy. Int J Radiat Oncol Biol Phys 1994;29:755–761.

19a. Beard CJ, Propert K, Clark J, et al. Complications after treatment with external beam irradiation in early stage prostate cancer patients: a prospective multi-institutional outcomes study. J Clin Oncol: In press.

20. Forman JD, Kumar R, Haas G, et al. Neoadjuvant hormonal downsizing of localized carcinoma of the prostate: effects on the volume of normal tissue irradiation. [See comments.] Cancer Invest 1995;13:8–15.

21. Johansson JE, Adami HO, Andersson SO, et al. High 10-year survival rate in patients with early, untreated prostatic cancer. JAMA 1992;267:2191–2196.

22. Chodak GW, Thisted RA, Gerber GS, et al. Results of conservative management of clinically localized prostate cancer. N Engl J Med 1994;330:242–248.

23. Porter AT, Blasko JC, Grimm PD, et al. Brachytherapy for prostate cancer. CA 1995;45:165–178.

24. Blasko JC, Ragde H, Grimm PD. Transperineal ultrasound-guided implantation of the prostate: morbidity and complications. Scand J Urol Nephrol Suppl 1991;137:113–118.

25. Nag S, Owen JB, Farnan N, et al. Survey of brachytherapy practice in the United States: a report of the Clinical Research Committee of the American Endocurietherapy Society. Int J Radiat Oncol Biol Phys 1995;31:103–107.

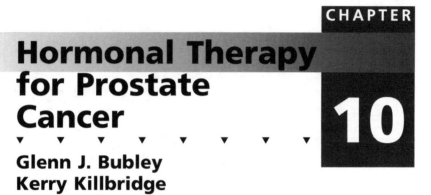

Hormonal Therapy for Prostate Cancer

CHAPTER 10

Glenn J. Bubley
Kerry Killbridge
Paul A. Church

SINCE THE pioneering work of Huggins more than 50 years ago, the cornerstone of treatment for metastatic prostate cancer has been hormonal therapy (1,2). Hormonal therapy is something of a misnomer, because what Huggins and his colleagues discovered was that *reducing* androgenic hormones, through the use of estrogens or by castration, is an effective therapy for many patients with metastatic prostate cancer (1). Since their discovery, for the past half century the therapy of choice for metastatic prostate cancer has been eliminating testosterone production by the testes (termed in this chapter either androgen deprivation or androgen ablation). Although androgen ablation is still a mainstay of therapy, recent scientific progress has resulted in a greater understanding of how the hormonal environment affects prostate cancer. These advances have led to newer hormonal therapies and applications, including novel methods of achieving androgen ablation and enhancing the utility of this therapy with the addition of other hormonal agents, such as antiandrogens. In addition, there is renewed interest in the timing of hormonal therapy, particularly in earlier stages of disease, including prior to and just after primary therapy of prostatic cancer. Insights into how prostate cancer cells survive in the androgen-depleted environment,

The authors wish to thank Drs. Steven Balk and Mary Anne Fenton for reviewing this chapter in manuscript form. Glenn J. Bubley dedicates this chapter to the memory of H. J. Bubley, a teacher and friend.

and why the disease recurs following hormonal therapy, have led to other hormone-based trials for this later stage of the disease. Clinical trials are even under way to determine if altering the hormonal environment in healthy men can prevent prostate cancer.

Because hormone-based clinical trials are rapidly evolving in the field of prostate cancer treatment, there are several current therapeutic trends that are not yet standard therapy but may prove to be useful. In this chapter, we will discuss the basic conceptual framework underlying the interaction between prostate cancer cells and the hormonal environment, thereby providing the basis for understanding future developments in this field.

■ ANDROGENS IN THE DEVELOPMENT OF THE NORMAL AND MALIGNANT PROSTATE GLAND

Androgens are the most important hormones for prostate growth and development (3). These hormones are not only crucial for the development of the normal prostate, but they also play a pivotal role in the development of prostate cancer. For example, in many animal models, the administration of large amounts of testosterone is required for the development of prostate cancer (3). Underscoring this laboratory observation is the fact that it has long been maintained that eunuchoid men do not develop this disease.

Androgens mediate growth and development in the prostate through a protein receptor located in the cytoplasm, called the androgen receptor (AR) (4–7). The AR is a member of the steroid superfamily of hormone receptors (5). Like its relatives, it has three general domains, including a carboxyterminal hormone- or ligand-binding domain, an aminoterminal transactivation domain, and a DNA-binding domain located between these regions (4–7). Following binding of the androgen to the hormone-binding domain, the receptor translocates to the nucleus, where the DNA-binding and transactivation domains are responsible for activation of a number of key genes involved in prostate growth and development (5,7). The importance of the AR in the development of the prostate is underscored by the effect mutations that inactivate the AR in individuals with the androgen-insensitivity syndrome (AIS). In this inherited syndrome, affected individuals fail to develop normal genitalia, including prostates (8), even in the presence of normal levels of androgenic hormones (7,8).

The main sources of androgens are the testes, which predominately synthesize testosterone (9). However, testosterone is readily converted in the prostate to 5-alpha-dihydrotestosterone (DHT) by the enzyme 5-alpha-reductase. DHT is more potent than testosterone by virtue of the fact that it has a higher affinity for the androgen receptor (10). Men who have a rare inherited defect in 5-alpha-reductase have smaller prostates and may be protected against prostate cancer (10–12). This observation, coupled with other laboratory insights, has contributed to the genesis of an ongoing hormonal prostate cancer prevention trial. The goal of this randomized trial is to prevent prostate cancer by decreasing the amount of DHT present in the prostate through the use of an inhibitor of 5-alpha-reductase, finasteride.

Testosterone is produced in the testes by Leydig cells. Leydig cells are stimulated to produce testosterone by the peptide, luteinizing hormone (LH), released by the pituitary (9). LH production is, in turn, under the control of luteinizing hormone–releasing hormone (LH-RH) (9,12). There is a direct interaction between LH-RH, LH, and testosterone production, and this hypothalamic-pituitary-gonadal interaction (Fig. 10.1) forms the basis of the androgen-ablative therapies discussed below. Importantly, testosterone and other steroid hormones, such as estrogen, are negative-feedback stimuli for LH-RH production (9,12).

There are multiple methods of achieving androgen ablation for the purposes of treating prostate cancer. However, all therapies have a common goal: reducing, by as much as possible, levels of serum testosterone. Following testosterone reduction, many normal cells and a vast majority of cancerous prostate cells follow a multigene-encoded "suicide pathway" called programmed cell death, or apoptosis (13). There is a population of normal prostate cells, and perhaps some prostate cancer cells, that do not die after androgen deprivation (14). The biologic nature of the hormone-resistant or androgen-independent cells is not certain. However, because the clinical response to androgen deprivation is always finite, it has been proposed that the "hormone-refractory cells" form the nidus of cells that re-

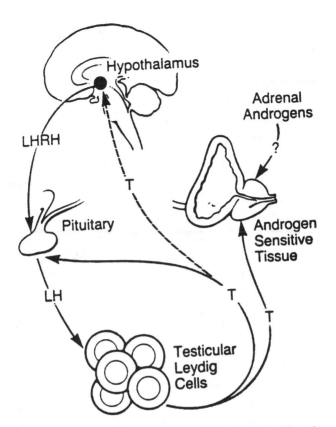

Fig. 10.1 *The hypothalamic-pituitary-gonadal axis. Pulsatile release of luteinizing hormone–releasing hormone (LH-RH) from the hypothalamus stimulates production of luteinizing hormone (LH) from the pituitary, which in turn stimulates production of testosterone (T) from Leydig's cells in the testes. In the prostate there are both normal and malignant cells that rely on testosterone, especially after conversion to 5-alpha-dihydrotestosterone (DHT), to stimulate growth. Adrenal androgens, especially if converted to T or DHT, are also likely growth stimulators. Testosterone and other hormones such as diethylstilbestrol (DES) inhibit the release of LH and LH-RH by a negative-feedback mechanism. (Reproduced by permission from McConnell JD. Physiologic basis for endocrine therapy for prostatic cancer. Urol Clin North Am 1991;18:1–13.)*

populate the bone marrow or other metastatic sites during relapse (15,16). An important area of current research is directed toward understanding how some prostate cancer cells are able to survive androgen deprivation.

■ EFFECTIVENESS AND METHODS OF ANDROGEN ABLATIVE THERAPY

A majority of patients with metastatic prostate cancer will respond to androgen deprivation therapy. However, the exact efficacy of this therapy is not known, because of the difficulty in assessing clinical response in this disease. In approximately 80% to 85% of patients, bone is the only site of metastasis (15). Since responding bone metastases typically only very slowly resolve on bone scan or plain films, it is problematic to objectively quantify response. Although about 15% of patients have sites of evaluable soft-tissue disease, often these sites are involved either late in the course or in patients with a less typical and more aggressive form of disease (15). Therefore it might not be possible to extrapolate the response rate of hormonal therapy from the responses of this patient subset.

With the recent introduction of prostate-specific antigen (PSA) measurements, the problem of objectively quantifying therapeutic response has improved (17). In most but not all cases, reductions in PSA have been shown to correspond to objective responses when studied in those patients who have evaluable bidimensional disease (17,18). Its conceivable that PSA measurements also reflect a measure of the androgen status of the cell, rather than strictly a measure of tumor burden. This is because PSA expression in controlled by an upstream regulatory DNA sequence that is activated when the androgen receptor is complexed to androgen (3). Levels of overall and prostate-specific fraction of acid phosphatase, and levels of alkaline phosphatase, are also useful for monitoring the status of the disease and the response to hormonal and other therapies (15).

With these caveats, most studies of androgen deprivation demonstrate objective response rates of 50% to 70% and even higher subjective response rates (80% to 90%) (15,16). Response rates are not usually affected by the particular method of androgen ablative therapy. Patients who tend to not respond to therapy have a greater frequency of visceral disease, and their tumors may have a less common neuroendocrine histology (19). In addition, lower serum testosterone and hemoglobin levels, lower performance scores, elevated acid and alkaline phosphatase levels, and greater degrees of bone involvement have all been shown to be independent negative prognostic variables (20–22).

Unlike the use of estrogen and progesterone levels in treating breast cancer, it is not standard practice to measure androgen receptor levels to predict the response to androgen deprivation therapy in prostate cancer. This is because efforts to retrospectively analyze AR levels and correlate these data have been mostly disappointing (23,24). Tests of AR expression are hampered because prostate cancer specimens, unlike breast cancer specimens, are almost always admixed with stromal and normal tissue. Because androgen ablative therapy has a high overall response rate and chemotherapeutic alternatives are relatively ineffective, predictive androgen receptor measurements may be less necessary in this disease than receptor measurements are for breast cancer.

Independent of the method of achieving androgen ablation, therapy usually results in an approximately 12- to 18-month duration of response (25–30). Because androgen ablative therapies induce prostatic cancer regression by the same mechanism, similar response rates and similar periods of response duration are not surprising. As will be discussed in the next section, the addition of antiandrogen therapy may lengthen the duration of response for some patients.

While it is the conviction of most clinicians that hormonal therapy results in an overall survival advantage, the evidence to support this assumption is not absolutely convincing. The pioneer trials of hormonal therapy for this disease started by the Veterans Administration Cancer Urologic Research Group (VACURG) employed a crossover option for placebo-treated patients, making it difficult to determine whether the hormonal therapy used in those studies resulted in a statistical survival advantage. Since that time, though few studies have utilized an untreated control arm, hormonal therapy has been generally shown to improve survival compared with historical controls.

The most simple method of reducing testicular androgens is

bilateral orchiectomy (27–30). This typically outpatient procedure is still the preferred method of therapy for many patients. One advantage this method has over other therapies is that it results in the almost immediate reduction of circulating androgens. Following orchiectomy, plasma testosterone is not measurable and does not increase, although LH levels rise and production of potentially important androgens from the adrenal gland continues (see below). Orchiectomy also has very low morbidity, its disadvantage being mostly psychological. Although orchiectomy is associated with loss of potency for many patients, it is often not appreciated that the other androgen ablative therapies typically result in impotency as well. Also similar to other androgen ablative therapies, orchiectomy can induce hot flashes (Table 10.1) and loss of muscle mass (27–30).

Along with orchiectomy, one of the first therapies for metastatic prostate cancer was diethylstilbestrol (DES), a synthetic estrogen preparation. Estrogens such as DES effectively lower testosterone by suppressing both the release and synthesis of LH-RH. Studies done in the 1940s and 1950s proved that estrogen was an effective therapy for prostatic carcinoma. In an important study published by Nesbit and Baum in 1950, it was concluded that, compared with historical controls, orchiectomy, DES, and the combination were associated with a longer survival in locally advanced disease (31). DES was formally compared with orchiectomy and placebo in the landmark cooperative group studies of the 1960s and 1970s. The first VACURG study published in 1967 involved more than 1,700 patients and compared placebo with bilateral orchiectomy, 5.0 mg of DES, and with orchiectomy plus DES (32). Importantly, this study showed that DES at the 5.0-mg level was associated with a significant increase in potentially life-threatening cardiovascular and thromboembolic complications. Finally, the combination of orchiectomy and DES did not prove to the superior to either one alone (32). The second VACURG study published in the early 1970s involved a randomized study of placebo compared with DES at doses of 0.2, 1.0, and 5.0 mg per day. This study showed that the 1.0-mg dose was as effective as the 5.0-mg dose in preventing cancer deaths but had significantly fewer cardiovascular complications. Long-term follow-up showed a trend toward improved overall survival in patients receiving the 1.0-mg dose of

Table 10.1 *Side Effects of Hormonal Therapy*

	Impotence	Hot flashes	Gynecomastia	Tumor flare	GI disturbance	Cardiovascular
Orchiectomy	++	+	+/–	–	–	–
DES	++	+	+/–	–	+	+
LHRH-A	++	++	+/–	+	–	–
Flutamide	–	++	+	–	+	–
Bicalutamide	–	++	+	–	–	–
Finasteride	–	–	–	–	–	–

(–) = rare; + = uncommon; ++ = common. Cardiovascular consists of thromboembolic events and edema for DES. GI disturbances are nausea and/or vomiting for DES and diarrhea for Flutamide.

DES (33). The third VACURG study also utilized the 1.0-mg dose of DES as a standard of comparison, comparing it with medroxyprogesterone acetate (Provera), conjugated estrogens (Premarin), and the combination of DES and medroxyprogesterone acetate. There were no significant survival differences in this study (34). In a comparable investigation, 1.0 mg of DES resulted in survival data similar to those obtained by orchiectomy or the combination of orchiectomy and the antiandrogen cyproterone acetate (35).

Although DES is still used for treating metastatic prostate cancer, it is used less frequently today than it was in the past. This is chiefly because of its significant thromboembolic risks and the introduction of LH-RH analogs (discussed below). DES also induces fluid retention and a painful gynecomastia (16,36), preventable by prophylactic chest irradiation.

The administration of other steroid hormones will also suppress LH production. These include conjugated estrogens, progesterones such as medroxyprogesterone acetate, and even androgens. However, each has significant side effects, and in general their efficacy has not been as well investigated as the other forms of androgen depleting therapy. Furthermore, due to the general acceptance of LH-RH analogs, these forms of therapy are not being widely investigated at present.

An increasingly popular method of reducing serum testosterone is the administration of depot injections of analogs of LH-RH (37). To understand how LH-RH analogs result in inhibition of testicular synthesis of testosterone, it is necessary to understand the nature of native LH-RH. The pituitary is stimulated to release LH by exposure to pulsatile amounts of LH-RH (3,9,12). In contrast, chronic LH-RH exposure actually blunts the pituitary response to this peptide, resulting in decreased release of LH. The LH-RH analogs used in clinical practice, such as leuprolide acetate and goserelin acetate, resemble the decapeptide they mimic (37,38). But the analogs have slight structural modifications (Fig. 10.2) that result in a peptide that has a much longer half-life than native LH-RH (gonadotropin-releasing hormone). Because LH-RH analogs so closely resemble native LH-RH, immediately after the initial injection there is stimulation of LH secretion resulting in a short period of higher than normal

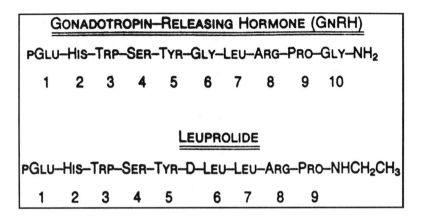

Fig. 10.2 *Comparison of gonadotropin-releasing hormone and the LH-RH analog leuprolide. The amino acid residues are similar in the peptides gonadotropin-releasing hormone, also known as luteinizing hormone–releasing hormone (LH-RH), and one of the LH-RH analogs, leuprolide. (Reproduced by permission from Garnick M, Glode LM, Smith JA, Leuprolide Study Group. Leuprolide vs diethylstilbestrol for metastatic prostate cancer. N Engl J Med 1984;311:1281–1286.)*

levels of testosterone (39). This initial period of administration had been associated with a tumor flare that can be ameliorated with concomitant antiandrogen administration (discussed below). Approximately two weeks after the initial injection, testosterone drops to very low levels, which persist during the entire course of therapy (26,37–39).

When LH-RH analogs were first developed, they had to be given by daily subcutaneous injection or intranasally, and the need to train patients or family members to administer this therapy diminished their acceptance. However, the development of monthly subcutaneous (goserelin acetate) and intramuscular (leuprolide) depot preparations made this unnecessary, and injections capable of lasting three months are now available. The main advantage of LH-RH agonists is the psychological benefit of not having to undergo orchiectomy. LH-RH agonists are also usually reversible, in that with discontinuation there can be recovery of the hypothalamic-pituitary-gonadal axis, and secretion of testosterone. This is a distinct advantage in clinical investigations that focus on the effect of relatively short-term androgen deprivation (approximately six months) prior to definitive therapy (see below). In the treatment of metastatic disease, reversibility is usually not necessary, and stopping LH-RH analog therapy may be ill-advised, even in relapsing patients. Some investigators have noted a flare in the disease with discontinuation of LH-RH analogs in relapsing patients, but this has not been confirmed in all studies (40,41). A disadvantage of LH-RH analogs is their cost. Monthly drug costs and administration charges can mount up quickly over the course of therapy.

The effectiveness of LH-RH analogs compared with other androgen suppressive therapies has been investigated in several well-performed studies. The Leuprolide Study Group showed that leuprolide acetate—at the time, administered daily—was as effective as 3 mg of daily DES for the treatment of D2 prostate cancer (26). However, leuprolide therapy was associated with fewer side effects. The only side effect reported at a greater frequency in the leuprolide group was hot flashes, while the DES group demonstrated a greater frequency of gynecomastia, nausea and vomiting, edema, and, most concerning, thromboembolism (27). Goserelin acetate has been compared with orchiectomy in a phase III randomized trial in the United Kingdom. The results were equivalent for rates of response (70%), time to progression, and survival (42). Based on these and other studies, it is generally accepted that LH-RH analogs are as effective as any other form of androgen ablative therapy, and are generally very well tolerated (42,43).

The side effects of common androgen ablative and antiandrogen therapies are listed in Table 10.1. LH-RH analogs, in addition to the antiandrogen therapy (discussed below), are associated with a slightly higher frequency of hot flashes than orchiectomy. Recently it has been shown that megesterol acetate is more effective than clonidine hydrochloride in ameliorating hot flashes (44). However, the effect on long-term tumor control of hormonal agents such as progesterone used in combination with androgen ablative therapies has not been investigated.

■ ANDROGENS AND TOTAL ANDROGEN BLOCKADE

As discussed above, with the initiation of LH-RH analog therapy, a minority of patients may experience an acute increase in pain at sites of bone involvement. These tumor flare responses are of particular concern if they lead to an exacerbation of cryptic cord compression. A number of studies demonstrated that antiandrogens can effectively ameliorate the tumor flare responses associated with rising testosterone levels after initial LH-RH analog injections (39). Antiandrogens, such as flutamide, seem to act by competing with androgens for the AR by occupying and blocking the receptor from the effects of stimulatory androgenic hormones. Testosterone falls to very low levels within the first month of therapy (37–39), reducing concern for flare responses and ostensibly eliminating the need for further antiandrogen therapy.

In the 1970s some investigators wondered whether there might be another role for antiandrogen therapy in the treatment of metastatic prostate cancer. They hypothesized that in patients treated with typical hormone therapy, the adrenal gland might serve as a source of hormones that allow prostatic cancer to grow and survive. Actually, this possibility was raised by Huggins and Scott in the early 1950s (45) as a rationale for bilateral adrenalectomy or hypophysectomy in relapsing orchiectomized patients. Responses to these surgical procedures were noted in some patients, perhaps validating their hypothesis. But the side effects of these procedures were very significant, and they largely fell out of favor.

The concern for adrenal stimulation of prostate cancer cell growth is related to the levels of adrenal androgens in hormonally treated patients. Synthesis of steroid hormones by the adrenals is largely under the control of adrenocorticotropic hormone (ACTH) from the pituitary, and the pituitary-adrenal axis is still functional in most patients. Although the adrenal synthesizes mainly glucocorticoids, this gland also synthesizes lesser amounts of androgenic hormones. The androgens released by the adrenal are predominantly dehydroepiandrosterone (DHA), dehydroepiandrosterone sulfate (DHAS), and androstenedione (3,9,46). These are only weak agonists of the AR by themselves, but they are potent stimulators depending on their peripheral conversion into testosterone and DHT in prostatic cancer cells (7,9). There is evidence that the enzymes necessary to convert these adrenal androgens into testosterone and DHT are present at significant levels in the prostate (7,9,10). Therefore, although castration results in a 90% reduction in serum testosterone levels, some investigators estimate that androgen levels may be reduced to only 60% in prostatic tissue (46). Furthermore, nonprimate animal models are not useful for determining the effect of adrenal hormones on prostate cancer biology, since castration in other species results in relatively complete androgen elimination (7). It is known that adrenal androgens are insufficient by themselves to induce prostate growth in an orchiectomized patient, but growth is possible after ACTH stimulation.

Adding to this complexity is the fact that even levels of circulating androgens are subject to change. The bulk of androgens in the circulation are complexed to sex hormone–binding globulins (SHBGs) and cannot bind to the AR (7). However, SHBG levels deviate widely depending on a number of systemic conditions, resulting in variations in the amount of free and bound androgen.

In this confusing theoretical background, the effects of antiandrogens in combination with androgen ablative therapy were studied in clinical trials started in the 1970s and 1980s. The first test of combination therapy, reported in 1979, was a negative study of the effect of cyproterone acetate and orchiectomy compared with orchiectomy alone (35). There was no improvement in duration of response or survival in patients treated with the combination therapy. However, Labrie and colleagues (47) investigated an antiandrogen more effective than cyproterone acetate, flutamide, in this patient population. In the mid-1980s they reported that flutamide significantly increased the time to progression and overall and disease-free survival compared with LH-RH analog therapy alone (47). A randomized prospective trial sponsored by the National Cancer Institute (NCI) under the leadership of Dr. E. D. Crawford (48) reported a statistically significant improvement in progression-free survival (16.5 versus 13.9 months) and overall survival (35.6 versus 28.3 months) in patients treated with the combination of leuprolide acetate and flutamide compared with leuprolide alone (Table 10.2). The European Organization for the Research and Treatment of Cancer (EORTC) compared orchiectomy with goserellin acetate and flutamide in a study started in 1985 (49). This study, published in 1993, also reported an improvement in overall survival for patients treated with combination therapy (Table 10.2). Other well-performed studies have not demonstrated a statistical survival advantage for combination therapy (50,51) (Table 10.2). Perhaps one reason for these discrepant findings is patient selection. Some studies have shown that the survival advantage for combination therapy is of greatest benefit for patients with lesser disease burdens, such as those who have a better performance status and fewer bone lesions at the initiation of therapy (48).

Antiandrogens can be divided into those that have a steroid hormone structure and nonsteroidal compounds. Examples of the former are cyproterone acetate and megesterol acetate, the latter include flutamide, nulitamide, and bicalutamide. Most studies of combination therapy have used flutamide or nilutamide as the antiandrogen. However, studies with a newer antiandrogen, bicalutamide (Casodex), show that, combined with an LH-RH analog, this once-a-day agent is perhaps as effective (52). As discussed above, nonsteroidal antiandrogens may also be more effective than steroidal antiandrogens in clinical trials (34). The fact that different antiandrogens may have different effects in vivo is not surprising. These com-

Table 10.2 *Representative randomized trials of combined androgen ablative and antiandrogen therapy compared with androgen ablative therapy alone*

Study	No. Patients	Treatment	Median Time to Failure (mo)	Median Overall Survival (mo)
Crawford et al. (48)	603	leuprolide	13.9*	28.3*
		leuprolide + flutamide	16.5*	35.6*
Denis et al. (49)	327	orchiectomy	21.2*	28.8*
		goserelin + flutamide	44.2*	43.9*
Beland et al. (50)	174	orchiectomy	11.7	18.9
		orchiectomy + nilutamide	12.4	24.3
Boccardo et al. (51)	373	goserelin	12.0	32.0
		goserelin + flutamide	12.0	34.0

*Statistically significant.
Goserelin = goserelin acetate.

pounds all have unique structures and demonstrate different in vitro properties, such as in their ability to compete with DHT for the androgen receptor (53,54).

Because of the common side effect of impotence in androgen ablative therapy, there has been interest in the use of antiandrogens alone (monotherapy) for patients who are still potent. Monotherapy has been shown to be generally inferior to orchiectomy and to LH-RH analog administration (55), and there are still ongoing trials, such as of the combination of flutamide and the 5-alpha-reductase inhibitor finasteride. But regardless of the outcome of these studies, if responses to androgen ablative therapy are unaffected by prior antiandrogen administration, monotherapy may be a more frequently used therapeutic modality because of its potency-sparing attributes.

Antiandrogens do have some side effects common to androgen deprivation, including hot flashes and breast enlargement and tenderness (Table 10.1). Most are associated with breast enlargement, breast tenderness, and hot flashes. Also flutamide has been associated with diarrhea in approximately 15% of patients. Some patients may better tolerate this agent if they are treated with lactase replacement therapy, as the drug is formulated with a lactose base (55).

■ THE TIMING OF ANDROGEN ABLATIVE THERAPY

Recently there has been renewed interest in the use of androgen ablative therapy in earlier stages of prostate cancer—specifically, prior to the onset of obvious symptomatic metastatic disease. The timing of hormonal therapy still needs to be investigated by several cooperative oncology groups in multiple clinical settings. These settings include its use in patients who have capsular penetration (stage C) or nodal involvement (stage D1), either immediately after radiation therapy or prostatectomy (adjuvant therapy), or for a finite time period *prior* to definitive radiation therapy or prostatectomy (neoadjuvant therapy). The ultimate goal of these studies is to improve survival, although neoadjuvant therapy may have additional benefits as well.

The question of whether it is more efficacious to use adjuvant hormonal therapy prior to the onset of symptoms in patients either destined or very likely to have significant clinical disease is one that has perplexed physicians treating prostate cancer almost since its inception. The crux of this question is whether earlier therapy translates into a survival advantage or just delays relapse. This question is not trivial, because unless adjuvant therapy results in a significant increase in survival, the side effects of androgen depleting therapy, especially impotence, and its expense, might not warrant its use. Even D1 (node-positive) patients can be symptom free for a number of years prior to the onset of bone pain or other symptoms referable to metastatic disease. Therefore, the implication of adjuvant therapy is that asymptomatic patients will be subjected to side effects for a long period. Furthermore, to prove its effectiveness, studies of adjuvant hormonal therapy necessarily need to involve many patients over a long follow-up period, particularly because survival is the most valid end point.

Although there is no substitute for well-run clinical studies, possible insights into the still unresolved question of "early" hormonal therapy might be gleaned from animal models. Issacs and colleagues demonstrated a survival advantage from castration in a well-differentiated androgen-sensitive rat prostatic adenocarcinoma model only in animals bearing small (<3 cc) tumors (56). These studies suggest that hormonal therapy could have curative potential in patients bearing smaller tumor burdens.

Although there are several ongoing studies investigating the efficacy of adjuvant hormonal therapy, there has also been some investigation of this question in the past. In the first and second VACURG studies, patients on the placebo arm were treated with hormonal therapy at the time of tumor progression, permitting a comparison of early versus late therapy in stage C and D patients. In these studies, the initial overall assessment was that delayed therapy did not appear to compromise overall survival. These data, presented in the early seventies, resulted in a change in practice for many physicians, in that hormonal therapy was often delayed until the onset of obvious symptoms. However, in 1988 the VACURG data were reanalyzed, and it was concluded that younger patients with high-grade (Gleason 7–10) and stage D disease may derive a survival benefit from early therapy (57).

In addition to the VACURG data, nonrandomized studies exist that suggest that adjuvant therapy may improve survival. In 1985 van Aubel reported in an uncontrolled study that slightly less than half of 30 patients with D1 disease progressed after 45 months following treatment with orchiectomy (58). The median survival of historic controls is roughly estimated to be 36 months. Therefore, although subject to the usual caveats regarding patient selection and other problems of an uncontrolled study, the authors suggested that early therapy leads to a survival benefit (58). In another nonrandomized study, by Zincke and colleagues, D1 patients treated with orchiectomy and primary surgical therapy had a better survival rate than patients treated with surgery alone (59). The benefit of the combined therapy was greatest in patients with diploid tumors. There are also several nonrandomized, primarily hormonal studies in patients with D1 and D2 disease that seem to show a possible survival advantage (60–62). These investigations have spurred the need for more well-designed, randomized-controlled trials.

In addition to investigating the effect of earlier hormonal therapy in asymptomatic patients after radiation or surgical therapy, there has also been a great deal of interest in using LH-RH analogs for a limited time prior to potentially curative primary radiation or surgical therapy. As discussed above, the goal of this neoadjuvant therapy is also to control micrometastases and improve overall survival. But an additional aim of therapy is related to reducing the side effects and improving the outcome of radiation therapy or surgery. These intermediate end points, unlike survival, can be defined and analyzed in the short term. Studies have focused on such questions as whether neoadjuvant therapy reduces the size of the tumor, resulting in down-staging, or decreases blood loss or surgical morbidity. Theoretically, if neoadjuvant therapy resulted in significant down-staging, it would permit patients who initially were not surgical candidates to become effective candidates for radical prostatectomy. In cases in which radiation is used to treat the disease, the hope is to reduce the volume of disease prior to therapy and thereby improve local control.

Studies to date of the ability of neoadjuvant therapy to affect these parameters are inconclusive. A pilot study of neoadjuvant hormonal therapy prior to radical prostatectomy was not conclusive as to either the issue of down-staging or the ease of surgical therapy (63). A study from Belgium actually showed greate degrees of blood loss and more surgical complications in patients treated with neoadjuvant hormonal deprivation (64). Among the problems in interpretation of these studies is the fact that there is no agreement on the period of pretreatment androgen ablation, so that the duration of neoadjuvant treatment may vary from as little as six weeks to as much as nine months.

In the absence of a greater number of randomized control trials, the benefits of neoadjuvant, or adjuvant, hormonal therapy in stage C, D1, or asymptomatic D2 patients are still not clear. Furthermore, current androgen ablative therapies can have potentially important side effects, such as impotence. Therefore it is most strongly recommended that, whenever possible, patients be enrolled in trials aimed at answering these important questions.

As discussed above, an unusual form of "early" therapy for prostate cancer involves modulating the hormonal microenvironment to try to prevent this disease. If the large multi-institutional NCI-sponsored study shows that the 5-alpha-reductase inhibitor finasteride reduces the incidence of prostate cancer, it will set the stage for the use of this agent or other hormonal agents to prevent prostate cancer.

■ HORMONAL THERAPY AFTER ANDROGEN ABLATION

Unlike breast cancer, with prostate cancer it has generally been the experience that additional hormonal therapies are unsuccessful, even in patients who previously responded to androgen ablative therapy. This impression has been advanced in part because responses to orchiectomy after progression on LH-RH analog therapy, or vice versa, are uncommon (55). This is not surprising, because both of these therapies are thought to induce remissions by the same mechanism, suppression of testosterone production. Although it has been recommended that testosterone levels be checked in patients relapsing on androgen ablative therapy, only uncommonly are measurable levels detected. These usually occur in patients treated with either DES for long periods or with low doses of DES. If measurable levels of testosterone are present, salvage LH-RH analog therapy or orchiectomy is appropriate.

In a break with past experience, based on both recent clinical and laboratory studies, there is renewed interest in other hormonal therapies in patients progressing after the initial androgen ablation. In fact, this reassessment holds sufficient promise that the authors prefer the narrower term *androgen independent* (AI), instead of hormone refractory, for patients progressing after initial testosterone depletion.

One strategy for treatment of AI disease is to block the secretion of adrenal hormones that possibly support prostate cancer growth, either by themselves or by conversion to testosterone and DHT. At high doses ketoconazole, an antifungal, can block the synthesis of adrenal hormones by blocking the conversion of cholesterol to pregnenolone, resulting in reduced production of glucocorticoids, mineralocorticoids, estrogens, and adrenal androgens (65). Although ketoconazole has gastrointestinal and other difficult side effects, objective responses have been reported in about one-sixth of patients able to tolerate the medication. Perhaps twice that number have had disease stabilization (65). A related compound, called liarozole, may prove to be more effective than ketoconazole and better tolerated (65). Suppression of adrenal cortex hormone production is also mediated by aminoglutethimide. In fact, the administration of this agent is often referred to as inducing a medical adrenalectomy (66). Aminoglutethimide is difficult to tolerate, due to side effects including lethargy and rashes, but responses have been achieved in a minority of patients (66,67). Since most patients on adrenal suppressive therapy need to be on glucocorticoids, it is conceivable that responses are mediated not only by inhibition of adrenal hormone synthesis, but also by adrenal suppression due to feedback inhibition or even as a direct effect of glucocorticoid-AR interaction. Responses to glucocorticoid therapy have been reported (68).

Another strategy for treating AI prostate cancer is to block the AR from whatever stimulating hormones are present in the tumor microenvironment. Antiandrogens such as flutamide have been found to result in approximately a 15% objective response rate in AI patients (69). Large trials of bicalutamide (Casodex) in AI disease are pending; however, responses to this agent have also been documented (70; Bubley, personal communication).

Progesterones, such as megestrol acetate, have been used in AI disease, but objective responses are uncommon (71,72). Similarly disappointing has been tamoxifen citrate, which, although it has demonstrated activity in animal models, was proven to be largely ineffective in human trials (73).

Recently a new and fascinating aspect of therapy for AI disease has emerged. It has been recognized that approximately 40% to 50% of patients will have a clinical response to discontinuing antiandrogen. These antiandrogen-withdrawal responses are relatively short-lived, lasting only about six months (74). Not only is antiandrogen withdrawal a sometimes useful clinical manuever, but it is also important for past and future clinical trials. For instance, if this variable is not controlled, clinical trials in AI-disease might generate false-positive responses to investigational agents in patients who may have just stopped taking flutamide. Tumor responses have also been detected after discontinuing bicalutamide (75).

How might discontinuing an antiandrogen result in a tumor response? One current hypothesis focuses on the interaction of the antiandrogen with the AR. Perhaps the emergence or apparent regrowth of tumor cells after androgen ablation is due to the presence of an AR that is no longer sensitive to the lack of DHT. Studies executed by Bubley in collaboration with Balk and other colleagues demonstrated that a mutant AR was expressed in 5 of 10 metastatic AI tumor sites (76). Of interest is that AR mutations detected in this setting seem to have the effect of broadening the specificity of the receptor, such that it could now be stimulated in vitro by androstenedione (77) and nonandrogenic steroid hormones such as estradiol (76) and progesterone (76,77). Furthermore, some in vivo–derived mutant ARs are actually stimulated by flutamide in vitro (Bubley, personal communication), as if the antiandrogen might actually result in growth stimulation instead of receptor blockade. A credible molecular explanation for the flutamide withdrawal syndrome is that for some AR mutants antiandrogens are agonists. This is indeed the case for the only prostate cancer cell line that expresses an androgen receptor, LNCaP cells. These cells actually proliferate following flutamide administration (78). Neither the frequency of mutant receptors in AI disease nor their exact biologic significance is known with certainty. However, a number of independent laboratories have now detected mutations in the AR from specimens obtained from patients with AI prostate cancer, confirming the overall observation that AR mutations exist in this stage of the disease (76,77,79,80).

Although most of the prostate tumor cell lines that can be passaged for long term in laboratory culture do not express an AR, this is not the case in human disease. The AR is expressed, and may even be overexpressed, in many tumor specimens derived from AI patients (81). This suggests that AI tumor cells may still be dependent on a functioning AR, either a wild type or a mutant, for survival. Overexpression of the AR might result in increased sensitivity to low levels of androgen, so that even the low amount of DHT contributed by conversion from adrenal androgens, for instance, is sufficient to fuel tumor growth.

■ FUTURE DIRECTIONS

Similar to other late-stage malignancies, advanced-stage prostate cancer is quite heterogeneous with respect to genetic phenotype and biologic activity. Such a diverse entity represents a formidable target for therapy. However, at least partial sensitivity to hormonal stimulation for growth and survival remains a unifying principle of treatment, and forms the basis for not only past therapy but also possible future trials.

One exciting approach is the administration of hormonal agents with different targets of activity, similar to the combination exemplified by antiandrogen and androgen ablative therapy for hormone-sensitive disease. For example, simultaneously stopping flutamide and adding aminoglutethimide has resulted in a moderate response rate in one study of AI patients (82). Other potentially useful combinations might both inhibit adrenal synthesis and block androgen receptors. These combinations may have their greatest utility in earlier stages of disease, in the setting of a smaller tumor burden.

The combination of existing or newer chemotherapeutic agents with hormonal therapy is also of interest. Henry and Isaacs demonstrated some time ago that the institution of cyclophosphamide in conjunction with orchiectomy was more effective than either one alone for cure in an animal model of prostate cancer (83).

Intermittent, instead of continuous, androgen deprivation therapy may be useful in delaying the emergence of AI disease. Experiments using an animal model suggest that androgen dependence can be prolonged by intermittent cycles of androgen ablation followed by reexposure to androgens (84).

Although it has been known for more than 50 years that androgen ablative responses are not permanent, the mechanism of recurrent disease is still not known with certainty. It is not known how a cell normally dependent on androgenic stimulation can survive in its absence. Many possible mechanisms have been postulated, including autocrine and paracrine stimulation by a host of specific growth factors, expression of a gene product known to inhibit apoptosis, and loss of proteins involved in cell cycle control. A discussion of these possibilities is beyond the scope of this chapter. However, it is doubtful that simply biologic selection for cells that have an altered affinity to testosterone, due to either increased or altered AR function, will explain the entire problem of AI disease. Nonetheless, the often persistent AR expression by these cells presents scientists and clinicians with a target for intervention that should not be overlooked, at for least short-term therapy.

This chapter has discussed a portion of the evolution of hormonal therapy for prostate cancer. Current basic and clinical research suggests that there will be a number of future uses for both existing and new hormonal therapies for all stages of this disease. Furthermore, it is hoped that the emerging insights into the dependence of prostate cancer on hormonal stimulation for development will result in an intervention that effectively reduces the incidence of clinical disease.

Editorial Comment

As the authors point out, hormonal therapy for prostate cancer has been an area of debate since Huggins's landmark work more than half a century ago. It is therefore important to reiterate where there is consensus and where there is controversy.

First, the areas of consensus: it is generally agreed that all three modalities of testicular androgen ablation are therapeutically equivalent. That is, orchiectomy, luteinizing hormone–releasing hormone (LH-RH) analogs, and estrogens all achieve the same clinical response. As the authors state, each modality has separate advantages and disadvantages, which must be individualized to each patient.

In addition, it is also agreed that all patients who receive hormone treatment for prostate cancer will eventually become hormone independent. Strategies such as intermittent hormone therapy or combination therapy utilizing chemotherapeutic agents and androgen blockade are being studied, but at the present time it is unproven whether they increase length of survival.

Major areas of controversy regarding hormone therapy persist. First, it is not known whether early versus late institution of hormone therapy provides any objective survival advantage to the patient. As the authors explain, the early Veterans Administration Cancer Urologic Research Group (VACURG) data suggested that the timing of hormonal therapy did not influence survival. More recent data have caused rethinking of this issue, with more investigators favoring the idea that there is an advantage to early institution of hormone therapy. However, the reader must be aware that at the present time no persuasive data exist to resolve this controversy.

The second topic of debate is whether total (testicular and adrenal) blockade is therapeutically superior to testicular blockade alone. Doctors Bubley, Killbridge, and Church correctly emphasize that data exist to support both sides of this question.

The final area of dispute is whether hormonal agents used as adjuvant therapy add to the efficacy of radical prostatectomy or external beam radiation therapy. The reader should recognize that several preliminary studies examining this issue have not provided consensus, and at the present time it is unproven whether adjuvant hormonal therapy prior to radical surgery or radiation therapy has any benefit in the treatment of prostate cancer.

■ REFERENCES

1. Huggins C, Hodges CV. Studies on prostatic cancer: effect of castration, of estrogen and androgen injections on serum phosphatases in

metastatic prostatic carcinoma of the prostate. Cancer Res 1941;1:293–297.

2. Huggins C, Clark PJ. Quantitative studies on prostatic secretion II: the effect of castration and of estrogen injection on the normal and on the hyperplastic prostate gland of dogs. J Exp Med 1940;72:747.

3. Liao S. Molecular actions of androgens. In: Litwack G, ed. Biochemical actions of hormones. Vol. 4. New York: Academic Press, 1977:351–406.

4. Lubahn BD, Joseph DR, Sar M, et al. The human androgen receptor: complementary deoxyribonucleic acid cloning, sequence analysis and gene expression in prostate. Mol Endocrinol 1988:1265–1275.

5. Beato M. Gene regulation by steroid hormones. Cell 1989;56:335–344.

6. Jenster G, van der Korput HAGM, van Vroonhoven C, et al. Domains of the human androgen receptor involved in steroid binding, transcriptional activation, and subcellular localization. Mol Endocrinol 1991; 5:1396–1404.

7. Hiipakka RA, Liao S. Androgen physiology: androgen receptors and action. In: Degroot LJ et al., eds. Endocrinology. 3rd ed. Philadelphia: WB Saunders, 1995:2336–2351.

8. Marcelli M, Tilley WD, Wilson CM, et al. Definition of the human androgen receptor gene structure permits the identification of mutations that cause androgen resistance: premature termination of the receptor protein at amino acid residue 588 causes complete androgen resistance. Mol Endocrinol 1990;4:1105–1116.

9. McConnell JD. Physiologic basis for endocrine therapy for prostatic cancer. Urol Clin North Am 1991;18:1–13.

10. Thigpen AE, Silver RI, Guileyardo JM, et al. Tissue distribution and ontogeny of steroid 5-alpha-reductase isoenzyme expression. J Clin Invest 1993;92:903–910.

11. Imperato-McGinley J, Gautier T. Inherited 5-alpha-reductase deficiency in man. Trends Genet 1986;2:130–133.

12. Griffin JE. Male reproductive function. In: Griffin JE, Ojeda SR, eds. Textbook of endocrine physiology. New York: Oxford University Press, 1988:165.

13. Kyprianou N, Isaacs JT. Activation of programmed cell death in the rat ventral prostate following castration. Prostate 1989;15:233–251.

14. Isaacs JT, Kyprianou N. Development of androgen-independent tumor cells and their implication for the treatment of prostatic cancer. Urol Res 1987;15:133–138.

15. Hanks C, Myers C, Scardino P. Cancer of the prostate. In: DeVita VT Jr,

Hellman S, Rosenberg SA, eds. Cancer: principles and practice of oncology. 4th ed. Philadelphia: JB Lippincott, 1993:1073–1113.

16. Grayhack JT, Keeler TC, Kozlowski JM. Carcinoma of the prostate:
hormonal therapy. Cancer 1987;60:589–601.

17. Shultz PK, Kelley W, Begg C, et al. Post-therapy change in PSA levels
as a clinical trial endpoint in hormone-refractory prostatic cancer: a
trial with 10-ethyl-deaza-aminopterin. Urology 1994;44:237–242.

18. Seidman A, Scher H, Petrylak D, et al. Estramustine and vinblastine:
use of prostate specific antigen as a clinical trial endpoint for hormone
refractory prostate cancer. J Urol 1992;147:931–934.

19. Di Sant'Agnese PA. Neuroendocrine differentiation in carcinoma of
the prostate: diagnostic, prognostic and therapeutic implications. Cancer 1992;72:254–267.

20. Matzkin H, Perito PE, Soloway MS. Prognostic factors in metastatic
prostate cancer. Cancer 1993;72:3788–3792.

21. Ernst DS, Hanson J, Venner PM, Uro-Oncology Group of Northern
Alberta. Analysis of prognostic factors in men with metastatic prostate
cancer. J Urol 1991;146:372–376.

22. Chodak GW, Vogelzang NJ, Caplan RJ, et al. Independent prognostic
factors in patients with metastatic (stage D2) prostate cancer. JAMA
1991;265:618–621.

23. Trachtenberg J, Walsh PC. Correlation of prostatic nuclear and androgen receptor content with duration of response and survival following
hormonal therapy in advanced prostate cancer. J Urol 1982;127:466–
471.

24. Sadi MV, Walsh PC, Barrack ER. Immunohistochemical study of androgen receptors in metastatic prostate cancer: comparison of receptor
content and response to therapy. Cancer 1991;67:3057–3064.

25. Haapianen R, Rannikko S, Althan O. Comparison of primary orchiectomy with estrogen therapy in advanced prostate cancer. Br J Urol
1986;58:528–533.

26. Garnick M, Glode LM, Smith JA, Leuprolide Study Group. Leuprolide
vs diethylstilbestrol for metastatic prostate cancer. N Engl J Med
1984;311:1281–1286.

27. Kaisary AV, Ryan P, Turkes A, et al. Comparison between surgical
orchiectomy and LHRH analogue (Zoladex, ICI 118630) in the treatment of advanced prostate carcinoma: a multicentre clinical study.
Prog Clin Biol Res 1988;260:89–100.

28. Daneshagari F, Crawford ED. Endocrine therapy of advanced prostate
carcinoma of the prostate. Cancer 1993;71:1089–1097.

29. Catalona WJ. Management of cancer of the prostate. N Engl J Med 1994;331:996–1004.

30. Denis L. Prostate cancer: primary hormonal treatment. Cancer 1993; 71:1050–1057.

31. Nesbit RM, Baum WC. Endocrine control of prostatic carcinoma: clinical and statistical survey of 1,818 cases. JAMA 1950;143:1317–1320.

32. Veterans Administration Cooperative Urological Research Group. Carcinoma of the prostate: treatment comparisons. J Urol 1967;134:292–298.

33. Byar DP. The Veterans Administration Coooperative Urological Research Group's studies of cancer of the prostate. Cancer 1973;32:1126–1130.

34. Byar DP, Corle D. Hormone therapy for prostate cancer: results of the VACURG studies. NCI Monogr 1988;7:165–170.

35. Robinson MRG. Complete androgen blockade: the EORTC experience comparing orchiectomy versus orchiectomy and cyproterone acetate versus low-dose stilbestrol in the treatment of metastatic carcinoma of the prostate. In: Smith PH, Pavone-Macaluso M, eds. Management of advanced cancer of the prostate and the bladder. EORTC Genitourinary Group Monograph 4. New York: Alan R. Liss, 1988:101–110.

36. Hedlund PO, Gustafsson H, Sjorgren S. Cardiovascular complications of treatment with prostatic cancer with estramustine phosphate or conventional estrogen: a follow-up of 212 randomized patients. Scand J Urol Nephrol 1980;55:103–105.

37. Conn PM, Crowley WF Jr. Gonadotropin-releasing hormone and its analogues. N Engl J Med 1991;324:93–103.

38. Ahmann FR, Citrin DL, DeHaan HA, et al. Zoladex: a sustained release luteinizing hormone–releasing hormone analogue for the treatment of advanced prostate cancer. J Clin Oncol 1987;5:912–917.

39. Kuhn J-M, Billebaud T, Navratil H, et al. Prevention of the transient adverse effects of gonadotropin-releasing hormone analogue (buserlin) in metastatic prostate cancer by administration of an antiandrogen (nilutamide). N Engl J Med 1989;321:93–103.

40. Hussain M, Wolf M, Marshall E, et al. Effects of continued androgen-deprivation therapy and other prognostic factors on response and survival in phase II chemotherapy trials for hormone-refractory prostate cancer: Southwest Oncology Group report. J Clin Oncol 1994;12:1868–1875.

41. Taylor CD, Elson P, Trump DL. Importance of continued testicular

suppression in hormone refractory prostate cancer. J Clin Oncol 1993;11:2167–2172.

42. Griffiths K. Is there a best castration? Cancer 1993;72:3807–3809.

43. Rosenberg AG, von Eschenbach AC. Hormonal therapy for prostate cancer. Semin Surg Oncol 1990;6:71–76.

44. Smith JA. A prospective comparison of treatments for hot flushes following endocrine therapy for carcinoma of the prostate. J Urol 1994;152:132–134.

45. Huggins C, Scott W. Bilateral adrenalectomy in prostatic cancer: clinical features and excretion of 17-ketosteroids and estrogen. Ann Surg 1945;122:1031–1041.

46. Geller J. Rationale for blockade of adrenal as well as testicular androgens in the treatment of advanced prostate cancer. Semin Oncol 1985;12:28–35.

47. Labrie F, Dupont A, Belanger A. Complete androgen blockage for the treatment of prostate cancer. In: De Vita VT, Hellman S, Rosenberg SA, eds. Important advances in oncology. Philadelphia: JB Lippincott, 1985:193–200.

48. Crawford ED, Eisenberger MA, McLeod DG, et al. A controlled trial of leuprolide with or without flutamide in prostatic carcinoma. N Engl J Med 1989;321:419–424.

49. Denis LJ, Carneiro De Moura JL, Bono A, et al. Goserllin acetate and flutamide versus bilateral orchiectomy: a phase III EORTC trial (30853). Urology 1993;42:119–130.

50. Beland G, Elhilali M, Fradet Y, et al. Total androgen ablation: Canadian experience. Urol Clin North Am 1991;18:75–82.

51. Boccardo F, Pace M, Rubagotti A, et al. Goserllin acetate with or without flutamide in the treatment of patients with locally advanced or metastatic prostate cancer. Eur J Cancer Clin Oncol 1992;8:1093–1096.

52. Shellhammer P, Sharifi R, Block N, et al. A controlled trial of bicalutamide versus flutamide, each in combination with luteinizing hormone–releasing hormone analogue therapy, in patients with advanced prostate cancer: Casodex combination study group. Urology 1995; 45:745–752.

53. McLeod DG. Antiandrogen drugs. Cancer 1993;71:1046–1049.

54. Geller J. Basis for hormonal management of advanced prostate cancer. Cancer 1993;71:1039–1045.

55. Dawson NA. Treatment of progressive metastatic prostate cancer. Oncology 1993;7:17–29.

56. Isaacs JT, Coffey DS. Adaptation versus selection as the mechanism responsible for the relapse of prostatic cancer to androgen ablation therapy as studied in the Dunning R-3327-H adenocarcinoma. Cancer Res 1981;41:5070–5075.

57. Kozlowski JM, Ellis WJ, Grayhack JT. Advanced prostatic carcinoma: early vs late endocrine therapy. Urol Clin North Am 1991;18:15–24.

58. Van Aubel OG, Hoeskstra WJ, Schroeder FH. Early orchiectomy for patients with stage D1 prostatic carcinoma. J Urol 1985;134:292–294.

59. Zincke H, Bergstralh EJ, Larson-Keller BS, et al. Stage D1 prostate cancer treated by radical prostatectomy and adjuvant hormonal therapy: evidence for favorable survival in patients with DNA diploid tumors. Cancer 1992;70:311–323.

60. Smith PH, Parmer M. Adjuvant therapy in prostatic cancer. Cancer 1993;71:992–995.

61. DeKernion J, Neuwirth H, Stein A, et al. Prognosis of patients with stage D1 prostate carcinoma following radical prostatectomy with and without early endocrine therapy. J Urol 1990;144:700–703.

62. Servadio C, Mukamel E, Lurie H, et al. Early combined hormonal and chemotherapy for metastatic prostatic carcinoma. Urology 1983; 21:493.

63. Fair WR, Aprikian A, Sogani P, et al. The role of neoadjuvant hormonal manipulation in localized prostatic cancer. Cancer 1993;71:1031–1038.

64. Van Poppel H, Ameye F, Oyen R, et al. Neo-adjuvant hormonotherapy does not facilitate radical prostatectomy. Acta Urol Belg 1992;60:73–82.

65. Mahler C, Verhalst J, Denis L. Ketoconazole and liarozole in the treatment of advanced prostate cancer. Cancer 1993;71:1068–1073.

66. Chang AYC, Bennett JM, Pandya, et al. A study of aminoglutethimide and hydrocortisone in patients with refractory prostate cancer. Am J Clin Oncol 1989;12:358–360.

67. Younge J, Appel J, Bergsman K, et al. Prolonged remissions with aminoglutethimide in advanced prostate cancer. Proc Am Soc Clin Oncol 1992;11:211. Abstract.

68. Tannock I, Gospodarowicz M, Maekin, et al. Treatment of metastatic prostate cancer with low-dose prednisone: evaluation of pain and quality of life as pragmatic indices of response. J Clin Oncol 1989;7:590–597.

69. Fossa SD, Hosbach G, Paus E. Flutamide in hormone-resistant prostate cancer. J Urol 1990;144:1411–1414.

70. Liebertz C, Kelley WK, Theodoulou M, et al. High dose Casodex for prostate cancer: PSA declines in patients with flutamide withdrawal responses. Proc Am Soc Clin Oncol 1995;14:232. Abstract.

71. Daniel F, MacLeod PM, Tyrell CJ. Megesterol acetate in relapsed carcinoma of the prostate. J Urol 1990;65:275–277.

72. Patel SR, Kvols LK, Hahn RG, et al. A phase II trial of megesterol acetate or dexamethasone in the treatment of hormonally refractory advanced carcinoma of the prostate. Cancer 1990;66:655–658.

73. Torti FM, Lum BL, Lo R, et al. Tamoxifen in advanced prostatic carcinoma: a dose-escalation study. Cancer 1984;54:739–743.

74. Scher HI, Kelley WK. Flutamide withdrawal syndrome: its impact on clinical trials in hormone refractory prostate cancer. J Clin Oncol 1993;11:1566–1572.

75. Small EJ, Caroll PR. Postate-specific antigen decline after Casodex withdrawal: evidence for an antiandrogen withdrawal syndrome. Urology 1994;43:408–410.

76. Taplin M-E, Bubley GJ, Shuster T, et al. Mutation of the androgen-receptor in metastatic androgen-independent prostate cancer. N Engl J Med 1995;332:1393–1398.

77. Culig Z, Hobisch A, Cronauer MV, et al. Mutant androgen receptor detected in advanced stage prostatic carcinoma is activated by adrenal androgens and progesterone. Mol Endocrinol 1993;7:1541–1550.

78. Olea N, Sakabe K, Soto A, Sonnenschein C. The proliferative effect of antiandrogens on the human prostate cancer cell line LNCaP. Endocrinology 1990;126:1457–1463.

79. Gaddipati JP, MacLeod DG, Heidenberg HB, et al. Frequent detection of codon 877 androgen receptor mutation in the androgen receptor gene in advanced prostate cancers. Cancer Res 1994;54:2861–2864.

80. Suzuki H, Sata N, Watabe Y, et al. Androgen receptor mutations in human hormone refractory prostate cancer. J Steroid Biochem 1993;46:759–765.

81. Hobisch A, Culig Z, Radmayr C, et al. Distant metastases from prostatic carcinoma express the androgen receptor. Cancer Res 1995;55:3068–3072.

82. Sartor O, Cooper M, Wienberger M, et al. Surprising activity of flutamide-withdrawal, when combined with aminoglutethimide, in treatment of "hormone-refractory" prostate cancer. J Natl Cancer Inst 1994;86:222–227.

83. Henry JM, Isaacs JT. Relationship between tumor size and the curabil-

ity of metastatic prostate cancer by surgery alone or in combination with chemotherapy. J Urol 1988;139:1119.

84. Akakura K, Bruchovsky N, Goldenburg SL, et al. Effects of intermittent androgen suppression on androgen-dependent tumors: apoptosis and serum PSA. Cancer 1993;71:2782–2790.

Management of Hormone Refractory Prostate Cancer

11

Kerry Killbridge
Donald S. Kaufman

▼   ▼   ▼   ▼   ▼   ▼   ▼   ▼

T HE TREATMENT of metastatic prostate cancer is androgen ablative hormonal therapy. Chemotherapy is reserved for patients who have failed hormonal treatment, and the results have been universally disappointing. Once androgen ablative treatment fails, median survival is 6 to 12 months (1). Unfortunately, despite intensive studies and many clinical trials, no currently available chemotherapy regimen offers significant promise in the treatment of metastatic prostate cancer. Historically, objective response rates to cytotoxic therapy have been in the 7% to 10% range (2), though a greater percentage of patients may report a temporary improvement in symptoms. The apparent discrepancy between objective decrease in the extent of disease and symptomatic improvement is explained by the prevalence of bony metastases in late-stage prostate cancer. It is well documented that changes in a bone scan or plain film may lag many months behind improvement in symptoms or never reflect that improvement at all (3). Change in soft tissue disease can be measured by standard bidimensional criteria, but a minority of patients have tumors at these sites. Over the past few years, a decrease in prostate-specific antigen (PSA) and improved quality of life have been correlated with symptomatic improvement not captured by standard criteria. As a consequence, response rates are higher with some new agents, but comparisons with older studies are difficult to make.

The use of PSA as a study end point in conjunction with quality-of-life measures has refined the ability to assess response rates to new agents. Studies reported from the Memorial Sloan-Kettering Cancer Center indicate that PSA may be a sensitive indicator of response (4). One hundred ten patients were treated with one of seven different protocols for hormone refractory prostate cancer, with the finding that a greater than 50% reduction in PSA was associated with a significantly improved median survival compared with patients with a less than 50% PSA reduction (5). It appears that PSA reduction may be the most significant factor in predicting survival in hormone resistant prostate cancer.

The first therapies to be considered in the treatment of cancers refractory to initial hormonal treatment, such as orchiectomy, luteinizing hormone–releasing hormone (LH-RH) agonists, and antiandrogens, are several secondary hormonal manipulations. In patients whose initial therapy has included total androgen ablation with LH-RH analogs, orchiectomy, or diethylstilbestrol (DES) plus flutamide, the simplest treatment consists of flutamide withdrawal. Scher and Kelly reported a 29% response rate, 10 of 36 patients, measured by 50% or greater decline in PSA in patients treated with prior hormonal therapy. Pain relief paralleled decline in PSA in patients with symptoms. Further analysis showed that no patients who started with hormonal monotherapy, subsequently added flutamide at disease progression, and then had flutamide stopped, responded to the withdrawal. Only patients who had received total androgen ablation at the outset of treatment responded to the withdrawal of flutamide. The authors noted that many therapeutic trials for androgen-resistant disease required the discontinuation of flutamide before the addition of the trial agent and therefore may be mistakenly attributing response to the trial agent rather than to flutamide withdrawal (6). Shortly thereafter, Dupont and colleagues confirmed these findings (7). Forty patients with progressive disease after total androgen ablation underwent flutamide withdrawal. Seventy-five percent responded according to the criteria of the National Prostatic Cancer Project. PSA fell to less than 50% of baseline in all but one of the responders (7). The explanation of this effect invokes the development of androgen hypersensitive clones through the upregulation of androgen receptors in the setting of low androgen levels. Regardless of how the phenomenon occurs, treatment is simple and response is rapid. Therefore patients deserve a trial of flutamide withdrawal before more toxic alternative therapies are used.

Alternative hormonal manipulation for patients whose initial treatment has been hormonal monotherapy with orchiectomy, estrogen therapy, or gonadotropin-releasing hormone analog include corticosteroids, antiandrogens, and possibly ketoconazole. The theoretical basis for these maneuvers lies in the observation that approximately 20% to 30% of androgen activity that fuels the growth of prostate cancer cells appears to be from prostatic conversion of steroid synthesis that is adrenal in origin (8). It is believed that the growth of prostate cancer cells can be slowed by blocking adrenal production after decreasing hypothalamic-pituitary stimulation of androgen precursor synthesis with primary hormonal therapy.

Moderate success has been observed with corticosteroids. Tannock and colleagues reported a 32% response rate, 12 of 37 patients, to low-dose prednisone at 5 mg twice a day, using pain and quality-of-life indices. Five patients who reported measurable improvements in pain and quality of life underwent reassessment of their disease with either bone scan or skeletal x-rays. Two showed improvement, 1 was unchanged, and 2 patients had deterioration of bone scans or x-rays. Unfortunately, only 7 patients reported improvement for longer than three months. Nonetheless, therapy was well tolerated, with only 1 patient reporting nausea and another reporting gastrointestinal pain (9). Similarly, Harland and Duchesne noted a 53% response rate, 8 of 15 patients, to hydrocortisone at 20 mg twice a day, as measured by a greater than 50% fall in serum PSA. Four additional patients experienced pain relief associated with a decrease in serum PSA to less than 80% of baseline. Median duration of response was six months (10). Older studies assessing change in measurable disease parameters without addressing symptomatic relief or decrease in serum PSA generally demonstrate lower response rates. Despite this difference, it is clear that corticosteroid therapy is a well tolerated and sometimes effective secondary hormonal therapy.

For patients who have not responded to hormonal monotherapy, the addition of flutamide appears to offer another secondary hormonal manipulation, with a substantial ability to palliate progressive disease. Labrie and colleagues reported a 34.5% response rate, 72 of 209 patients, to the addition of flutamide after treatment with orchiectomy, LH-RH analogs, or DES. Response was assessed by change or stabilization of measurable disease according to the criteria of the National Prostatic Cancer Project. Patients receiving DES were switched to LH-RH analogs, and patients already receiving LH-RH analogs were continued on therapy while flutamide was added to their regimen. Median life expectancy was greater than 30 months for responders versus 8.1 months for nonresponders. At least 6.2% of patients demonstrated a complete response. Overall, 80% of patients reported hot flashes and 8% suffered gastrointestinal side effects, but no patients required discontinuation of therapy (8). Because flutamide addition is so well tolerated and easy to administer, it presents an attractive treatment alternative to corticosteroids as secondary hormonal therapy. Bicalutamide, similar in activity and mechanism of action to flutamide, is a new addition to the available hormonal treatments in the therapy of metastatic prostate cancer. There are data that suggest that in doses of equal therapeutic efficacy, patients experience fewer gastrointestinal side effects than with flutamide (11).

Both ketoconazole and aminoglutethimide were studied as secondary treatments for progressive prostate cancer in the 1980s. As mentioned previously, the theoretical basis for their use was total androgen blockade by inhibiting adrenal steroid synthesis after gonadal synthesis has been blocked with orchiectomy, DES, or LH-RH analogs. A high rate of clinical adrenal insufficiency observed with these drugs necessitates the concomitant use of corticosteroids. As evidence grew that steroids alone can result in a substantial response, it became unclear whether results once attributed to ketoconazole and aminoglutethimide were due to these agents or to the corticosteroids with which they were administered. A mounting body of laboratory evidence supports adrenal gonadal suppression secondary to corticosteroids rather than aminoglutethimide (12,13). As a result, it would appear that there is little role for this agent after first-line hormonal therapy. The use of ketoconazole is less clear. At least one study that examined PSA response to ketoconazole and prednisone noted that 12 of 15 patients experienced a drop of more than 38% in PSA, and 75% of patients, 9 of 12, with bone pain reported improvement in symptoms (14). Since some of this response is probably due to prednisone, it is unclear how much benefit can be credited to ketoconazole. It is difficult to recommend ketoconazole over other secondary hormonal therapies with a well-defined response. This drug has also been used with other agents. A recent study combining ketoconazole with doxorubicin has documented a 55% response rate using PSA to measure efficacy. Severe mucositis, stomatitis, and neutropenia were observed, requiring hospitalization of 45% of patients in the study. Sixty-three percent of patients received corticosteroid therapy for clinical adrenal insufficiency (15). Although some of the response rate may be due to ketoconazole and doxorubicin, the severe toxicity and confounding use of corticosteroids do not warrant use of this combination off protocol. In a similar study, medroxyprogesterone acetate (Provera) was used in combination with epirubicin for hormone refractory cancer. Di Leo and colleagues treated 54 patients with 1,000 mg of daily medroxyprogesterone acetate combined with weekly epirubicin, 30 mg/m^2. Of 23 patients with measurable disease, 26% had an objective partial response to therapy, but 52% of the 54 patients had a 50% or greater decrease in their analgesic requirement. Three patients suffered clinically significant cardiac toxicity, reversible at the discontinuation of therapy. Other common side effects included nausea, myelosuppression, and alopecia. Although the combination of epirubicin and medroxyprogesterone acetate provided relief of symptoms in a significant number of patients, the mean duration of response was only four months and median survival was not prolonged over that achieved with supportive care (16). These agents continue to warrant investigation, but the results to date are not encouraging.

After secondary hormonal maneuvers have been exhausted, cytotoxic chemotherapy may be considered in the treatment of hormone refractory tumors. Standard response criteria that gauge a bidimensional decrease in measurable disease have frequently underestimated the subjective improvement reported by patients enrolled in chemotherapy trials. Using a 50% or greater decrease in PSA as the major criterion, a few single agents have demonstrated consistent response rates with minimal toxicity. Oral cyclophosphamide (Cytoxan) has been shown to produce a response rate of approximately 30% by this standard, with a significant decrease in pain in at least two single-institution trials. Abele and colleagues treated 20 patients with 100 mg/m of daily oral cyclophosphamide for two weeks every 28 days and observed a 30% response rate measured by PSA decrease of 50% or more (17). Similarly, von Roemeling and colleagues noted a 31% response rate in 13 patients who received a total daily dose of 75–150 mg (18). Patients in both trials had been heavily pretreated with other chemotherapeutic agents, hormonal manipulations, and radiation therapy. Toxicity side effects were predominantly mild myelosuppression that did not require hospitalization or transfusion, and nausea, controlled with antiemetics. Higher dose intravenous cyclophosphamide alone or in combination with other agents has been associated with more toxicity without demonstrable advantage.

Mitoxantrone also appears to be a promising single agent, despite the fact that in early studies doxorubicin, a related anthracycline, had been shown to have little activity in hormone refractory prostate cancer (19). In addition, this agent produces less nausea, vomiting, alopecia, and cardiotoxicity than doxorubicin. Mitoxantrone hydrochloride has reproducibly demonstrated a response rate of approximately 30% in several small pilot and phase II studies using a variety of dosing regimens. Moore and colleagues treated 27 patients with mitoxantrone, 12 mg/m^2 IV every 3 weeks, and daily low-dose prednisone. He noted a response rate of 36% using quality-of-life measures that surveyed pain and social functioning (20). Knopf and colleagues treated 10 patients with weekly doses of 10 mg/m^2 and observed a 50% or greater reduction in PSA in 30% of patients (21). Kantoff and associates treated 15 patients with a 14-day continuous infusion of 1.0–1.5 mg/m^2/day mitoxantrone every 28 days, and demonstrated a 33% subjective improvement but only a 13% decrease in PSA of 50% or greater (22). Trials of combination chemotherapy with mitoxantrone have resulted in increased toxicity without appreciable benefit.

Many other single agents have been studied with disappointing results. Despite activity in germ cell tumors, cisplatin, carboplatin, and etoposide produce little response in hormone refractory prostate cancer. Three different phase II studies of cisplatin, 50–70 mg/m^2 every three weeks, demonstrated a less than 20% partial response rate measured by a greater than 50% tumor reduction or a decrease by more than 50% in acid phosphatase level (23–25). Although a pilot study suggested an improved 43% response rate with weekly dosing, these results were not confirmed by subsequent phase II evaluation conducted by Moore and colleagues. Their Southeast Cancer Study Group trial administered 40 mg/m^2/week for six weeks, followed by 60 mg/m^2 every three weeks to 33 patients. Only 3 patients had normalization of alkaline or acid phosphatase and no patients had regression of measurable disease, resulting in a response rate of 10% (26). Single-agent carboplatin given weekly at 150 mg/m^2 failed to improve these results. Cannobio and colleagues studied this regimen in 25 patients with hormone refractory prostate cancer and noted a 17% partial response rate (27). Etoposide was found to have even less activity than platinum-based therapy in several phase II trials using similar response criteria. Walther and colleagues treated a group of 36 patients with 130 mg/m^2 etoposide, daily for 3 days every 21 days, and noted only one partial response (28). Scher and associates used a slightly lower dose, 100 mg/m^2, on the same schedule and documented only one partial response (29). At least one study conducted by Trump and Loprinzi has investigated a continuous infusion schedule for etoposide. No objective response was seen in 20 patients who received 50 mg/m^2/day for 5 days every 28 days (30).

Methotrexate, 5-fluorouracil, and paclitaxel (Taxol) have also been used as single agents in hormone refractory prostate cancer. All three drugs have proven ineffective. Murphy and the investigators of the National Prostatic Cancer Project studied methotrexate at 40 mg/m^2 on day one, 60 mg/m^2 on day six and every two weeks thereafter, in 52 patients (31). They observed partial regression of measurable disease in only 1 patient. Similarly, minimal benefit was documented in regimens of 5-fluorouracil as a bolus infusion. As a result, the Illinois Cancer Center examined 5-fluorouracil given as a continuous infusion, 1,000 mg/m^2/day for 5 days every 28 days in a phase II trial of 25 patients. No objective responses were observed. Cardiac toxicity was significant, including one sudden death, one episode of supraventricular tachycardia, and one episode of congestive heart failure (32). Despite its remarkable activity in other malignancies, paclitaxel produces little response in hormone refractory prostate cancer. Roth and colleagues administered paclitaxel as a 24-hour continuous infusion at 135–170 mg/m^2 every 21 days to 23 patients in an Eastern Cooperative Oncology Group (ECOG) phase II trial. Although 1 patient experienced a partial response, toxicity was severe. Fever and neutropenia developed in 6 patients, and three cardiovascular events were documented, including two sudden deaths (33). In short, toxicity has far outweighed any marginal benefit derived from single agent cytotoxic chemotherapy for most drugs except cyclophosphamide and mitoxantrone.

Unfortunately, almost all combination chemotherapies result in more frequent and more extreme toxicities than single-agent regimens for hormone refractory prostate cancer, and benefits have been marginal. Combinations with estramustine appear to be the exception. Two regimens with estramustine appear to have significant activity without prohibitive side effects. The structure of estramustine is an estradiol linked to a nornitrogen mustard. Estramustine appears to inhibit microtubule formation, in addition to working at the level of the nuclear matrix. As a single agent, estramustine has little activity in prostate cancer cell lines, but preclinical studies documented compelling evidence for synergy between estramustine and etoposide or vinblastine sulfate (34). These results led Hudes and colleagues to conduct a phase II evaluation. The investigators treated 36 patients with oral estramustine 600 mg/m on days 1 through 42, and vinblastine sulfate 4 mg/m IV weekly for six weeks, and documented that 61% of patients had a decrease in PSA of greater than 50% and a marked improvement in painful metastases. Only three episodes of grades 3 to 4 leukopenia were observed (35). In an effort to create a completely oral regimen, Pienta and associates (36) treated 42 patients with an oral regimen of estramustine 15 mg/m/day and oral etoposide 50 mg/m/day in daily divided doses. Overall, 52% of patients experienced a 50% or greater reduction in PSA. Of 18 patients with measurable soft tissue disease, 3 patients had a complete response and 6 patients had a partial response, for a 50% response rate by standard criteria. Myelosuppression was much more severe than observed with the vinblastine sulfate combination, leading to five episodes of fever and neutropenia and one death from bone marrow failure (36). Early results with combination regimens using estramustine are encouraging, but randomized multi-institutional trials will be necessary to confirm the initial response rates and to determine whether there is any survival benefit over single agents or supportive care.

Once patients have begun chemotherapy, it is unclear whether they should continue to be treated with androgen suppression. Two retrospective analyses have addressed the issue, with conflicting results. Taylor and colleagues reviewed four ECOG trials of various chemotherapies and found that ongoing androgen suppression was a statistically significant predictor of survival in a Cox multivariate analysis that included performance status, weight loss, disease site, and prior radiation therapy. The differences in median survival were modest depending on the trial, from two to six months, but the investigators recommended careful consideration before discontinuing androgen suppression (37). Hussain and colleagues reviewed pooled results of six Southwestern Oncology Group (SWOG) phase II trials of different cytotoxic regimens. His group found no survival difference between patients who continued androgen suppression versus those who stopped hormonal treatment while undergoing chemotherapy (38). Both studies were retrospective, with small numbers of patients who had discontinued androgen suppression. Unfortunately, the answer to the question of whether to continue androgen suppression with chemotherapy will probably require prospective investigation. For patients who decide to enter a chemotherapeutic trial, the decision to continue androgen suppression can be tailored to entrance criteria and treatment protocol.

In addition to standard cytotoxic drugs, two experimental therapies have generated a great deal of enthusiasm in the treatment of hormone refractory prostate cancer. Both suramin sodium and bone-seeking radiopharmaceuticals appear to have novel antitumor mechanisms with promising response rates. Suramin is a polysulfonated naphthylurea developed in the 1920s to treat the trypanosome responsible for African sleeping sickness. In the past few years the drug has been used to treat hormone refractory prostate cancer. The antitumor effect of suramin was thought to result from its ability to bind growth factor receptors and interrupt their stimulation of tumor progression. With further study it has become evident that suramin binds kinase-binding proteins, inhibits reverse transcriptase, and induces transforming growth factor alpha, all of which may be involved in the drug's antitumor activity. Meyers and colleagues published one of the first studies of this novel compound. The group treated 38 patients with hormone refractory prostate cancer and found that 55% experienced a drop in PSA of 50% or more. Of 13 patients with a 75% or more decrease in PSA, 85% were alive at one year. Several patients were alive close to two years after treatment, suggesting that there may ultimately be a survival benefit to treatment. In 17 patients with measurable soft tissue disease, 3 patients had complete regression of all detectable disease and 3 patients had a partial response. These encouraging results have to be weighed against the considerable toxicity of the compound. Bleeding disorders, adrenal insufficiency, rash, renal insufficiency, and myelosuppression with infection were all documented in 30% or more of patients. Most troublesome, however, was a sensorimotor polyneuropathy that sometimes progressed to a Guillain-Barré syndrome, requiring respiratory support and resulting in patient death (39). The neurologic toxicity of suramin sodium is significantly decreased by maintaining plasma levels below 300 μg/mL, but the other side effects remain. The long half-life, 55 days, and narrow therapeutic window required intensive monitoring of plasma drug levels with early regimens. More recent fixed-dose regimens appear to maintain drug levels well within the therapeutic range without the necessity of monitoring plasma levels (40,41). The response rates observed in suramin treatment clearly deserve further investigation in protocol studies.

Strontium-89, samarium-153, and rhenium-186 comprise the other experimental therapies in addition to suramin that have shown promise in the treatment of hormone refractory prostate cancer. Because the drugs are taken up by bone, they preferentially localize to blastic metastatic sites in prostate cancer and deliver a higher dose of radiation to the area of metastatic disease than to normal bone. All three agents have proven effective in providing pain relief in 50% or more of patients in numerous small trials (42–44). Despite symptomatic relief, there is rarely any objective evidence of tumor regression by PSA or other criteria. Strontium-89 is the best studied of the three drugs. Overall, pain relief takes one to three weeks after injection but may be accompanied by a flare in symptoms in 10% to 20% of patients before any clinical improvement occurs. Other side effects include mild, transient thrombocytopenia. Relief may persist for up to six months and can be followed with retreatment. At least two trials suggest that treatment with strontium-89 versus local radiotherapy may delay development of new painful bony metastases for several months after treatment (45,46). Although toxicity appears to be minimal in comparison with suramin, there are no long-term survivors after treatment with strontium. The impressive pain relief obtained with radiopharmaceuticals supports further trials, but they are still considered experimental treatments and should be used only in investigational protocols.

In summary, hormone refractory prostate cancer usually declares itself with a rising PSA during treatment with initial hormonal therapy. No treatment for progressive disease has yet been proven to prolong survival. As a result, there is no standard chemotherapeutic regimen in this situation. Young patients with little comorbid disease and good performance status will better tolerate the side effects of cytotoxic chemotherapy or other experimental regimens, and these patients should be considered for treatment on protocol as early as possible. Given the toxicity of even low-dose oral chemotherapy without clear improvement in survival, chemotherapy off protocol is not recommended. Local radiation therapy can provide pain relief at specific sites and is useful in the treatment of impending pathologic fractures. This therapy should be used as needed in conjunction with other modalities. Finally, despite the encouraging results with suramin, a few chemotherapeutic agents, and the newer radiopharmaceuticals, these therapies all remain experimental and require further investigation before they can be recommended as standard treatment.

Editorial Comment

In this chapter the authors comprehensively review the subject of hormone insensitive prostate cancer. It is important to realize that from a patient's perspective, the most meaningful end points for treatment are quantity and quality of life. No treatment for hormone refractory prostate cancer has been shown to be life prolonging; however, significant palliation can be achieved with a variety of therapies.

A reasonable approach to systemic therapy for symptomatic patients would be:

1. Withdrawal of antiandrogen (flutamide or bicalutamide)
2. Alternative hormonal therapy (ketoconazole, aminoglutethimide, steroids)
3. Chemotherapy

Chemotherapy should be considered for patients in whom the potential benefits of palliation outweigh the risks of toxicity.

Radiation in the form of external beam radiation or radiopharmaceuticals are useful adjuncts. Symptom management with pain medications, stool softeners, and psychosocial support are critical.

New drugs and approaches are sorely needed. Thus, patients should be encouraged to enter in clinical trials.

■ **REFERENCES**

1. Sellers W, Kantoff PW. Nonhormonal therapy for hormone-refractory prostate cancer. In: Yalla S, Loughlin KR, eds. Benign and malignant diseases of the prostate. New York: Plenum, 1992.
2. Yagoda A, Petrylak D. Cytotoxic chemotherapy for advanced hormone-resistant prostate cancer. Cancer 1993;71(suppl):1098–1109.
3. Scher HI, Yagoda A. Bone metastases: pathogenesis, treatment, and rationale for use of resorption inhibitors. Am J Med 1987;82:6–28.
4. Redman BG, Pienta KJ. New treatment strategies for hormone refractory prostate cancer. Semin Urol 1995;13:164–169.
5. Kelly WK, Scher HI, Mazumdar M, et al. Prostate-specific antigen as a measure of disease outcome in metastatic hormone-refractory prostate cancer. J Clin Oncol 1993;11:607–615.
6. Scher HI, Kelly WK. Flutamide withdrawal syndrome: its impact on clinical trials in hormone-refractory prostate cancer. J Clin Oncol 1993;11:1566–1572.
7. Dupont A, Gomez J-L, Cusan L, et al. Response to flutamide withdrawal in advanced prostate cancer in progression under combination therapy. J Urol 1993;150:908–913.

8. Labrie F, Dupont A, Giguere M, et al. Benefits of combination therapy with flutamide in patients relapsing after castration. Br J Urol 1988;61:341–346.

9. Tannock I, Gospodarowicz M, Medkin W, et al. Treatment of metastatic prostatic cancer with low-dose prednisone: evaluation of pain and quality of life as pragmatic indices of response. J Clin Oncol 1989; 7:590–597.

10. Harland SJ, Duschesne GM. Suramin and prostate cancer: the role of hydrocortisone. Eur J Cancer Clin Oncol 1992;28:1295.

11. Schellhammer P, Sharifi R, Block N, et al. A controlled trial of bicalutamide versus flutamide, each in combination with luteinizing hormone–releasing hormone analogue therapy, in patients with advanced prostate cancer. Urology 1995;45:745–752.

12. Plowman PN, Perry LA, Chard T. Androgen suppression by hydrocortisone without aminoglutethimide in orchiectomised men with prostatic cancer. Br J Urol 1987;59:255–257.

13. Dowsett M, Shearer RJ, Ponder BAJ, et al. The effects of aminoglutethimide and hydrocortisone, alone and combined, on androgen levels in post-orchiectomy prostatic cancer patients. Br J Cancer 1988;57:190–192.

14. Gerber GS, Chodak GW. Prostate specific antigen for assessing response to ketoconazole and prednisone in patients with hormone refractory metastatic prostate cancer. J Urol 1990;144:1177–1179.

15. Sella A, Kilbourn R, Amato R, et al. Phase II study of ketoconazole combined with weekly doxorubicin in patients with androgen-independent prostate cancer. J Clin Oncol 1994;12:683–688.

16. Di Leo A, Bajetta E, Buzzoni R, et al. Epirubicin plus medroxyprogesterone as second-line treatment of advanced prostatic cancer. Am J Clin Oncol 1995;18:239–244.

17. Abele FL, Wilkes JD, Divers L, et al. Oral cyclophosphamide for hormone refractory prostate cancer. Proc Am Soc Clin Oncol 1995;243.

18. Von Roemeling R, Fisher HAG, Horton J. Daily oral cyclophosphamide is effective in hormone refractory prostate cancer: a phase I/II study. Proc Am Soc Clin Oncol 1992;213.

19. Torti FM, Shortcliffe LD, Carter SK, et al. A randomized study of doxorubicin versus doxorubicin plus cisplatin in endocrine-unresponsive metastatic prostatic carcinoma. Cancer 1995;56:2580–2586.

20. Moore MJ, Osoba D, Murphy K, et al. Use of palliative endpoints to evaluate the effects of mitoxantrone and low-dose prednisone in

patients with hormonally resistant prostate cancer. J Clin Oncol 1994;12:689–694.

21. Knopf R, Knopf K, Ganesh L, et al. Pilot study of low dose weekly mitoxantrone as a single agent in widely metastatic hormone-refractory prostate cancer. Proc Am Soc Clin Oncol 1993:250.

22. Kantoff PW, Bryant P, Block C, et al. Fourteen day constant infusion of mitoxantrone HCL for hormone refractory carcinoma of the prostate: a pilot dose study finding. Proc Am Soc Clin Oncol 1991:175.

23. Yagoda A, Watson RC, Natale RB, et al. A critical analysis of response criteria in patients with prostatic cancer treated with *cis*-diaminedichoride platinum II. Cancer 1979;44:1553–1562.

24. Qazi R, Khandekar J. Phase II study of cisplatin for metastatic prostatic carcinoma. Am J Clin Oncol 1983;6:203–205.

25. Rossof AH, Talley RW, Stephans R, et al. Phase II evaluation of *cis*-dichlorodiamineplatinum (II) in advanced malignancies of the genitourinary and gynecologic organs: a Southwest Oncology Group Study. Cancer Treat Rev 1979;63:1557–1564.

26. Moore MR, Troner MB, DeSimone P, et al. Phase II evaluation of weekly cisplatin in metastatic hormone-resistant prostate cancer: a Southeastern Cancer Study Group trial. Cancer Treat Rev 1986;70:541–542.

27. Cannobio L, Guarneri D, Miglietta L, et al. Carboplatin in advanced hormone refractory prostatic cancer patients. Eur J Cancer 1993;29:2096–2100.

28. Walther P, Williams SD, Troner M, et al. Phase II study of etoposide for carcinoma of the prostate. Cancer Treat Rev 1986;70:771–772.

29. Scher HI, Sternberg C, Heston WDW, et al. Etoposide in prostatic cancer: experimental studies and phase II trial in patients with bidimensionally measurable disease. Cancer Chemother Pharmacol 1986;18:24–26.

30. Trump DL, Loprinzi CI. Phase II trial of etoposide in advanced prostate cancer. Cancer Treat Rev 1984;68:1195–1196.

31. Murphy GP, Priore RL, Scardino PT, et al. Hormone-refractory metastatic prostatic cancer treated with methotrexate, cyclophosphamide plus adriamycin, *cis*-platinum plus 5-fluorouracil plus cyclophosphamide. Urology 1988;32:33–40.

32. Kuzel TM, Tallman MS, Shevrin D, et al. A phase II study of continuous infusion 5-fluorouracil in advanced hormone refractory prostate cancer. Cancer 1993;72:1965–1968.

33. Roth BJ, Yeap BY, Wilding G, et al. Taxol in advanced, hormone-refractory carcinoma of the prostate. Cancer 1993;72:2457–2460.

34. Pienta KJ, Lehr JE. Inhibition of prostate cancer growth by estramustine and etoposide: evidence for interaction at the nuclear matrix. J Urol 1993;149:1622–1625.

35. Hudes GR, Greenberg R, Krigel RL, et al. Phase II study of estramustine and vinblastine, two microtubular inhibitors, in hormone-refractory prostate cancer. J Clin Oncol 1992;10:1754–1761.

36. Pienta KJ, Redman B, Hussain M, et al. Phase II evaluation of oral estramustine and oral etoposide in hormone-refractory adenocarcinoma of the prostate. J Clin Oncol 1994;12:2005–2012.

37. Taylor CD, Elson P, Trump DL. Importance of continued suppression in hormone-refractory prostate cancer. J Clin Oncol 1993;11:2167–2172.

38. Hussain M, Wolf M, Marshall E, et al. Effects of continued androgen-deprivation therapy and other prognostic factors on response and survival in phase II chemotherapy trials for hormone-refractory prostate cancer: a Southwest Oncology Group report. J Clin Oncol 1994;12:1868–1875.

39. Meyers C, Cooper M, Stein C, et al. Suramin: a novel growth factor antagonist with activity in hormone-refractory metastatic prostate cancer. J Clin Oncol 1992;10:881–889.

40. Reyno LM, Egorin MJ, Eisenberger MA, et al. Development and validation of a pharmacokinetically based fixed dosing scheme for suramin. J Clin Oncol 1995;13:2187–2195.

41. Kobayashi K, Vokes EE, Vogelzang NJ, et al. Phase I study of suramin given by intermittent infusion without adaptive control in patients with advanced cancer. J Clin Oncol 1995;13:2196–2207.

42. Curley T, Scher H, Thaler H, et al. (Re-186-HEDP) for palliation of painful bone metastases from prostatic cancer. Proc Am Soc Clin Oncol 1991:347.

43. Turner JH, Claringbold PG, Hetherington EL, et al. A phase I study of samarium-153 ethylenediaminetetramethylene phosphate therapy for disseminated skeletal metastases. J Clin Oncol 1989;7:1926–1931.

44. Robinson RG, Preston DF, Spicer JA, et al. Radionuclide therapy of intractable bone pain: emphasis on strontium-89. Semin Nucl Med 1992;22:28–32.

45. Bolger JJ, Dearnaley DP, Kirk D, et al. Strontium-89 (Metastron) versus external beam radiotherapy in patients with painful boney metastases

secondary to prostatic cancer: preliminary report of a multicenter trial. Semin Oncol 1993;20:32–33.

46.   Porter AT, McEwan AJB, Powe JE, et al. Results of a randomized phase-III trial to evaluate the efficacy of strontium-89 adjuvant to local field external beam irradiation in the management of endocrine resistant prostate cancer. Int J Radiat Oncol Biol Phys 1993;25:805–813.

Diet and Nutrition in Prostate Cancer Prevention and Therapy

12

▼   ▼   ▼   ▼   ▼   ▼   ▼   ▼

Steven K. Clinton

DIET AND NUTRITION are relevant to three distinct stages of prostate cancer. First, the role of the foods, nutrients, and long-standing dietary patterns in the genesis of prostate cancer should be a concern of all men in the United States. In addition, we will soon be able to more precisely define prostate cancer risk based on familial associations and genetic markers. Men at greater risk will be motivated to alter lifestyle factors or participate in chemoprevention trials to prevent the development of prostate cancer. Although much more information is needed, general dietary guidelines and recommendations have been developed that are appropriate for prostate cancer prevention in American men, particularly those who are at high risk. A second area of interest concerns the role of diet and nutrition in men undergoing or having completed therapy for early-stage prostate cancer (organ confined or locally advanced) who are concerned about the possibility of future recurrent or progressive disease. This group of men frequently falls prey to purveyors of unproven, expensive, and potentially harmful diet and nutrition schemes. Providing sound dietary guidelines to these men may prevent many from pursuing alternative programs of questionable benefit. The third area of prostate cancer management in which sound nutritional support is needed involves the care of those suffering from metastatic disease, particularly those with the cachexia syndrome. These three areas of nutrition and prostate cancer will be reviewed separately.

■ DIETARY RECOMMENDATIONS FOR PROSTATE CANCER PREVENTION

The role of nutrition in the etiology of prostate cancer has not been thoroughly investigated, and much more information will be derived from ongoing epidemiologic and laboratory studies. Cancer of the prostate has become one the most frequently diagnosed cancers in American men, and it is especially common among the African-American population (1,2). It is estimated that prostate cancer is currently the fourth most common malignancy diagnosed in men worldwide. However, the incidence and mortality rates vary greatly according to geographic location, race, and ethnicity (2). The international distribution of prostate cancer is similar to that of colon and breast cancer, with higher age-adjusted incidence and mortality rates in North America and northern Europe (2) (Fig. 12.1). In contrast, many developing nations and Mediterranean countries have very low prostate cancer mortality rates. In addition, Japan, which has experienced significant economic development in recent decades, continues to exhibit very low rates of prostate cancer incidence and mortality. It has been suggested that these striking variations in the worldwide distribution of prostate cancer are due to differing genetic backgrounds. However, studies of populations that have migrated from low-risk areas to high-risk areas clearly show an increase in prostate cancer rates. For example, Chinese or Japanese migrants show an upward shift in age-adjusted prostate cancer risk on migrating to the United States (3). Similarly, African-American men exhibit a much higher rate of prostate cancer than African men (Fig. 12.2). These observations strongly support the hypothesis that some aspects of the environment, such as the diets of those in more affluent societies, may be very important in the etiology of prostate cancer.

Geographic and migrant studies have generated diet and prostate cancer hypotheses that are investigated in case-controlled, retrospective, and prospective epidemiologic studies focusing on diet and nutrition (4,5). In addition, laboratory investigations in rodent models and in vitro systems under precisely controlled conditions provide additional clues to the roles that diet and nutrition may play in the pathogenesis of prostate cancer (4,5). It is clear that no single

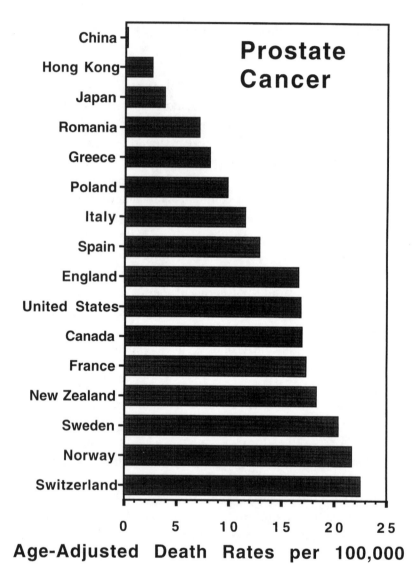

Fig. 12.1 *Worldwide distribution of prostate cancer (age-adjusted death rates per 100,000 men). (From Boring CC, Squires TS, Tong T, et al. Cancer statistics. CA 1994;44:7–26.)*

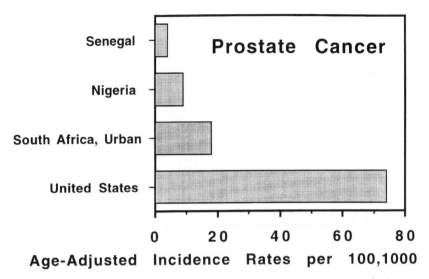

Fig. 12.2 *Prostate cancer in African-American men versus populations in Africa. (From Boring CC, Squires TS, Heath CW, et al. Cancer statistics for African Americans. CA 1992;42:7–18.)*

component of the diet is the primary cause of prostate cancer. Rather, a number of factors acting together in the affluent diet appear to be associated with the increased risk observed in our society. The dietary pattern as a whole is more critical than any single factor. Table 12.1 lists dietary guidelines that are appropriate for men in the United States, particularly those at risk of prostate cancer. These recommendations are based on current research in prostate cancer etiology and prevention and are similar to recommendations for cancer prevention derived from a number of sources, including the National Cancer Institute, the American Cancer Society, the National Research Council of the National Academy of Sciences, the United States Department of Agriculture, and the World Health Organization (6–10). At the present time, more than 90% of American men fail to meet or adhere to these readily achievable goals. Men and their families who are motivated to make changes in their diet but lack a basic understanding of diet and nutrition will benefit from the instruction and guidance of a registered dietitian. In addition, a few of

Table 12.1 *Ten dietary recommendations for prostate cancer prevention*

1. Maintain a healthy body weight through moderation in energy intake and regular physical exercise.
2. Choose a diet low in total fat, saturated fat, and cholesterol.
3. Increase consumption of fresh fruits and vegetables to at least five servings per day.
4. Increase consumption of complex carbohydrates and fiber from whole-grain cereals, breads, and pasta.
5. Consume meats in moderation and from diverse sources, including fish.
6. Use sugar and salt in moderation.
7. Drink alcoholic beverages in moderation.
8. Choose your diet based on the principles of variety, moderation, and balance.
9. Avoid nutrient supplements in excess of the RDA in any one day.
10. Avoid unproven and potentially dangerous alternative therapies, health products, and diet schemes.

the publications available in bookstores provide sound dietary and nutritional information (11,12).

Physicians should recognize that controversy exists within the scientific and medical community, food industry, and government regulatory agencies concerning the development of diet and nutrition guidelines to prevent cancer. Some argue that dietary changes should not be recommended until scientific uncertainties have been resolved. In contrast, many others believe that the associations observed justify efforts to change the American diet while more definitive data are obtained from ongoing investigations. Unfortunately, absolute proof for many of the diet and prostate cancer hypotheses will be very difficult, if not impossible, to obtain due to the expense required to complete long-term intervention studies in large numbers of subjects. The following recommendations take into account several factors, including strength of the scientific evidence, potential benefits from a reduced risk of prostate cancer as well as other diet-associated diseases, likelihood and severity of an adverse effect from the recommended change, and the feasibility of men achieving the desired goal. Although it is impossible to quantify the impact that these guidelines may have on prostate cancer risk, most experts agree that these recommendations can be made with a reasonable degree of certainty, with the likelihood of minimal risk, and the potential for significant public health benefits, including a decreased risk of prostate cancer (6–10).

1. Maintain a Healthy Body Weight Through Moderation in Energy Intake and Regular Physical Exercise: It is very difficult to dissect the complex interrelationships between total energy consumption, energy expenditure and exercise, change in body mass index, genetic differences in energy metabolism, and the risk of prostate or other cancers. However, increased body weight or obesity has been associated with prostate cancer risk in some, but not all, studies (4,5). In addition, data from an extensive array of carefully controlled studies in laboratory rodents suggest that excess energy intake enhances carcinogenesis of the prostate and other tissues (13). Excess weight is associated with increased risk of hypertension, hyperlipidemias, cardiovascular disease, adult-onset diabetes mellitus, and osteoarthritis. The increasingly sedentary American population continues to exhibit a rising mean body weight even while average total energy intake is stabilizing or slightly decreasing. Body weight is a balance between the energy consumed from the diet and the amount of energy used by normal metabolism and physical exercise. Even small differences between intake and expenditure can, over time, lead to appreciable differences in body weight. To loose weight, the individual must utilize, or "burn up," more calories than consumed by increasing exercise and eating less. Regular physical exercise should be a critical component of a weight loss program. It is well established that fad or crash diet programs can produce serious medical problems and are of little long-term value because the weight lost is quickly regained, a phenomenon known as "yo-yo" dieting. Many of the following dietary recommendations will contribute to a successful weight loss program, which should approximate one to two pounds per week.

2. Choose a Diet Low in Total Fat, Saturated Fat, and Cholesterol:
A diet rich in lipids, particularly saturated fats, as well as cholesterol
is characteristic of nations where prostate cancer is common. International and intracountry epidemiologic studies have suggested strong
associations between age-adjusted prostate cancer risk and the per
capita intake of total fat. Similarly, several analytical epidemiologic
studies, case-control studies, and recent cohort studies have reported
associations between prostate cancer risk and total fat intake, consumption of high-fat foods, or animal fat consumption (3,5,14–16). In
addition, some laboratory studies of prostate cancer support the
positive relationship between dietary fat and prostate cancer progression (17). The dietary fat and prostate cancer hypothesis will continue
to be evaluated in order to better define the mechanisms involved and
quantify the benefits to be derived from reducing fat intake. In addition to the possible role of high-fat diets in prostate cancer etiology,
accumulating evidence suggests a role for high-fat diets in cardiovascular disease as well as other cancers, such as those of the large bowel.
There is general agreement among the nutrition community that the
American diet is excessively rich in fats and cholesterol. Most expert
committees recommend reducing total fat intake to less than 30% of
calories, with saturated fats reduced to less than 10% of calories and
cholesterol limited to less than 300 mg/day (6–10,12). These goals can
be accomplished by substituting fish, poultry without skin, lean
meats, and low- or nonfat dairy products for fatty meats and whole-
milk dairy products, and by eating more fruits, vegetables, cereals,
and legumes, in conjunction with limiting fats and oils in cooking,
spreads, and dressings.

**3. Increase Consumption of Fresh Fruits and Vegetables to at Least
Five Servings per Day:** The consumption of fruits and vegetables is
associated with a reduction in cancer risk for many tissues, including
lung, larynx, esophagus, colon, stomach, pancreas, bladder, cervix,
ovary, and endometrium (18). Fruits and vegetables contribute in
many ways to a healthy diet. They have a lower caloric density and
contribute to satiety and a higher fiber intake. In addition, it is likely
that specific fruits and vegetables will prove to have unique protec-
tive effects for certain types of cancer. For example, it has been

hypothesized that the frequent consumption of tomatoes, tomato paste, and tomato sauce is associated with a reduced risk of prostate cancer (19). Although very speculative at the present time, the carotenoid lycopene, which provides the red color to tomato products, is currently being investigated for specific anti–prostate cancer properties (20). An understanding of which constituents in these foods have anticancer properties will lead to the development of food extracts or purified chemical components for chemoprevention studies in high-risk groups. Recognizing that the guideline of five servings per day is accomplished by fewer than 10% of Americans, the National Cancer Institute has initiated the "Five a Day for Better Health" program designed to help Americans increase their daily consumption of fruits and vegetables. The program also emphasizes that vitamin supplements do not provide the same health benefits as eating a variety of fruits and vegetables.

4. Increase Consumption of Complex Carbohydrates and Fiber from Whole-Grain Cereals, Breads, and Pasta: Approximately 55% to 60% of daily calories should be derived from carbohydrates, with an emphasis on complex carbohydrates derived from breads, cereals, pasta, rice, potatoes, and beans and other legumes (12). Like the fruits and vegetables, these foods provide fiber to prevent constipation and perhaps other bowel disorders, and they are associated with a reduced risk of cardiovascular disease. In addition, they have a lower caloric density and contribute to early satiety, which assists in maintaining energy balance and body weight.

5. Consume Meats in Moderation and from Diverse Sources, Including Fish: Several epidemiologic studies suggest that diets rich in red meat are associated with greater prostate cancer risk (16). However, the basis for this relationship remains very speculative. Perhaps men who have a diet rich in red meat also consume fewer fruits and vegetables or complex carbohydrates, as well as a high level of saturated fats. It has not been clearly established that a specific component of the meat per se is an initiator or promoter of prostate cancer. Efforts are under way to better understand the possible role of red meat in prostate carcinogenesis and how processing and cooking may be involved. In recent decades, the meat industry has been significantly reducing the amount of fat and cholesterol in meat products in response to consumer demand stimulated by the dietary fat–heart disease relationship. At the present time, a reasonable approach is to consume meats in moderation and to include seafood. There is no strong evidence suggesting that elimination of all meat products from the diet (vegetarianism) as a sole dietary intervention will have a significant impact on prostate cancer risk. A well-planned vegetarian diet can provide all of the nutrients necessary for health, but whether such a diet is more healthful compared with a diet that includes moderate meat intake has not been established. For those interested in a vegetarian approach, particularly one avoiding all meat and milk products, a consultation with a registered dietitian would be recommended to ensure that the diet provides a good balance of essential amino acids and adequate sources of vitamins D, B_{12}, and riboflavin, as well as the minerals calcium, iron, and zinc.

6. Use Sugar and Salt in Moderation: Sugar is not the evil agent responsible for the destruction of our physical and psychiatric health, as many food faddists have proclaimed (12). Sugar per se is not the cause of diabetes, heart disease, or cancer. Sugar is associated with tooth decay when one snacks frequently without thoroughly cleansing the teeth. The problem is that foods rich in sugar are often highly refined and devoid of other nutrients and natural substances that may have beneficial effects (12). In addition, foods rich in sugar are often teamed with fats in high-calorie foods such as candy, ice cream, and pastries. Therefore, sugar should be consumed in moderation in order to assist in meeting the overall dietary goals.

There is no evidence that salt intake is related to prostate cancer. In contrast, the evidence linking excess salt intake to hypertension, which contributes to the progression of cardiovascular disease, has been established. Salt intake should be limited to less than 6 gm/day, primarily by reducing its use in cooking and at the table.

7. Drink Alcoholic Beverages in Moderation: There is little evidence at the present time to implicate alcohol in prostate cancer. Overall, moderate consumption is not harmful for most people, and it may even be desirable for those at risk of cardiovascular disease. A moderate amount is defined as no more than one drink per day for women, and two for men. A drink is defined as 12 ounces of beer, 5 ounces of wine, or 1.5 ounces of liquor. In contrast, chronic overindulgence in alcohol is clearly harmful. Alcohol intake is strongly associated with cancers of the oropharynx, larynx, and esophagus, particularly when it is used in combination with tobacco products. Alcoholic beverages probably contribute to liver cancer and may have a role in gastric, pancreatic, colon, and breast cancer, although additional studies will be necessary to firmly establish and quantify risk for the latter malignancies. Chronic alcohol intake damages vital organs such as the liver and brain, contributes significantly to traffic fatalities, and is well known to increase birth defects when consumed during pregnancy. Alcoholic beverages are rich in calories and low in nutrients, thereby contributing to excess weight and reduced intake of various nutrients. Moderation in alcohol intake is a safe recommendation for overall health (12).

8. Choose Your Diet Based on the Principles of Variety, Moderation, and Balance: The key to a healthy diet is variety, moderation, and balance (12). These three terms are incorporated into the dietary recommendations and guidelines developed by numerous experts and committees in the area of diet, nutrition, and public health (6–10,12). Variety means avoiding repetitive meal patterns and selecting a diverse array of grains, fruits, vegetables, dairy, and meat items as meals are composed over time. Moderation in the consumption of any one food or nutrient avoids excess caloric intake and harmful excesses of nutrients. Balance is achieved by variety and moderation as well as by maintaining an equilibrium between calories consumed and energy expenditure.

9. Avoid Nutrient Supplements in Excess of the RDA in Any One Day: The purveyors of nutrient supplements have led Americans to mistakenly believe that supplementing is necessary and beneficial for the majority of otherwise healthy people. In reality, the notion that average Americans experience a "vitamin gap" or need supplements for "insurance" is a myth (11,12). Many Americans believe that the recommended daily allowance (RDA) for a nutrient is synonymous with a dietary requirement and that if you do not ingest the full RDA of a specific nutrient each day, your diet is somehow deficient. Health care providers should recognize that RDAs are set at the upper end of the normal distribution curve to ensure adequacy in nearly 95% of the population. Otherwise healthy men, adhering to the dietary guidelines presented in Table 12.1, will achieve adequate supplies of all known nutrients, including the vitamins and minerals. Below the RDAs, the intake levels that are minimally acceptable are not known with accuracy or precision for many nutrients and are not uniformly agreed on. One example for which there is sufficient knowledge is vitamin C. The average person requires no more than 10 mg of vitamin C per day to prevent scurvy. The RDA of 60 mg is sufficient to produce substantial body stores of vitamin C, while the average American consumes more than 70 mg from the diet. Millions of Americans consume megadoses of vitamin C in the mistaken belief that it prevents various ailments, despite the lack of objective studies supporting these claims. Megadoses of vitamin C are not harmless and can produce a number of problems, including diarrhea and occasionally metastatic oxalosis involving the kidney and heart.

Caregivers should recognize that most adults do not need supplements to prevent nutrient deficiencies. There are individuals in the population who are a higher risk of vitamin or mineral deficiencies, and physicians should provide dietary guidance and supplements to these individuals (12). Supplements are recommended during pregnancy and lactation, for example. Iron deficiency in menstruating women is a prevalent nutritional problem in Americans. Those who are socioeconomically disadvantaged, consume bizarre diets, or suffer form chronic alcoholism and other illnesses are at higher risk of nutrient insufficiencies and may benefit from counseling and nutritional support.

Many prostate cancer patients have read or been advised that supplementation with vitamins A, E, and C, and the mineral selenium may have beneficial effects with regard to prostate cancer. However, the research completed so far does not support beneficial effects of excessive supplementation with these substances. Evidence suggests a complex role for vitamin A, pro–vitamin A carotenoids, and synthetic retinoids in prostate carcinogenesis. In a series of studies, estimates of vitamin A intake have been reported to have no relationship or to be associated with increased or decreased risk of prostate cancer (4,19). A number of studies in laboratory models indicate that vitamin A deficiency (a condition that is very rare in Americans) increases the susceptibility of many tissues, including the prostate, to chemical carcinogens. However, these observations should not be used to support the belief that supplements may reduce risk in men who have an adequate vitamin A intake from their diet. Since the benefits of excess vitamin A intake are unsubstantiated and the potential for significant toxicity exists for the fat-soluble vitamins, it is wise to avoid supplements in excess of the RDA. The development of synthetic retinoids, which have unique effects within the prostate, is an exciting and rapidly evolving area of study that may lead to novel agents for chemoprevention trials in high-risk men.

Vitamin E is a supplement consumed by many who perceive that they are at risk of cancer or cardiovascular disease. Vitamin E is a family of eight compounds collectively referred to as tocopherols. Vegetable oils, eggs, dark green vegetables, and whole grains or legumes are the major sources of dietary vitamin E, and a deficiency syndrome has never been defined in humans. Nutritional scientists still do not fully understand the roles of vitamin E, and the optimal intake beyond that which prevents deficiency has not been established. The issue of potential health benefits from supplemental intake in excess of the RDA remains controversial. The antioxidant and free radical scavenger properties of vitamin E have suggested a possible role as an antineoplastic vitamin. However, the data derived from epidemiologic studies, rodent experimentation, and intervention studies have not provided strong evidence to support the consumption of vitamin E supplements to prevent prostate cancer. It is not clear how harmful chronic consumption of large doses of vitamin E may be to men, although moderate supplementation beyond the RDA of 10 μg seems to be tolerated.

Vitamin C functions as a general antioxidant and is a component of several enzymatic reactions in intermediary metabolism. Citrus fruits, leafy vegetables, tomatoes, and potatoes are rich sources of vitamin C. Despite the intense interest in vitamin C over recent decades, there is almost no evidence to support a role for vitamin C in the prevention of prostate or other cancers. At the present time the consumption of vitamin C supplements at levels significantly higher than can be achieved with a well-balanced diet or a multivitamin should be discouraged. Individuals consuming more than 1 gm of vitamin C per day are at risk of rebound scurvy if they discontinue supplements without a gradual tapering off.

The mineral selenium is an essential constituent of a cellular enzyme system called glutathione peroxidase, which participates in the destruction of hydrogen peroxide and organic hydroperoxides. Selenium, therefore, participates in cellular and tissue defense against oxidative damage and, perhaps, exogenous carcinogenic agents. Selenium in the diet from grains and cereals, mushrooms, onions, and garlic depends on the amount of the mineral in the soil. Chicken and seafood are also sources of selenium. Marginal selenium intake does not produce clear clinical symptoms, but reduced intake has been proposed to predispose to injury by various agents, such as certain chemical carcinogens. Overall, conclusions concerning a role for selenium in the prevention of human prostate cancer cannot be justified at this point in time. Supplementation of the diet beyond the RDA of 70 μg for men should be discouraged; the mineral has significant risk of toxicity beyond 200 μg/day.

An increasing proportion of the American population consumes some type of nutritional supplement on a daily basis. The public views supplementation as an important form of self-therapy for the prevention and treatment of many ailments, including cancer (11,12). Vitamin supplements are easy to consume, relatively free of side effects when consumed at RDAs, and can be obtained without a prescription. In addition, multivitamin and mineral supplements can be inexpensive, although the cost of many products is greatly inflated. One of the most attractive aspects of vitamin or mineral supplementation is the mistaken belief that the supplement may counteract the adverse effects of a poor diet or a lifestyle factor such as smoking, which is much more difficult to change. These issues emphasize the importance of scientifically sound studies to define the risks and benefits of nutrient supplements for the prevention of chronic diseases, such as cancer. Caregivers must recognize that many individuals with a diagnosis of cancer, or those concerned about the risk of cancer due to familial trends, genetic factors, or known environmental exposures to carcinogens, are readily persuaded by proponents of supplements. The multibillion dollar supplement industry includes health food stores, mail-order catalogs, and a diverse array of practitioners of "alternative" medicine. In reality, we must recognize that it is very difficult to educate patients and family members with regard to supplement use. A sensible approach with individuals who are taking supplements or who are inclined to take them is to guide them toward the use of a multivitamin and mineral supplement from a reputable supplier that approximates the RDAs. There is little risk involved in this approach, and it may prevent the consumption of potentially toxic amounts of other supplements.

10. Avoid Unproven and Potentially Dangerous Alternative Therapies, Health Products, and Diet Schemes: Cancer ranks as the second leading cause of death in affluent nations, and survival rates for major forms of cancer have not improved significantly, despite a large investment of public resources in research and health care. The perceived failure of the medical and scientific establishment to prevent and treat cancer has led the public toward unproven fads and remedies. Some of the well known and dubious alternative treatment methods include homeopathy, naturopathy, iridology, macrobiotic diet, orthomolecular therapy, psychic healing, colonic irrigation, crystal healing, and the consumption of "glandulars," enzymes, and herbal products (11,12,21). Americans spend billions on products and programs that allegedly have the power to prevent or reverse the process of aging and the development of chronic disease. In addition to being ineffective and potentially dangerous, these products and programs are invariably expensive. It is not enough for caregivers to point out the dangers. Persuading a person to abandon a fad diet or program involves providing a rational alternative that will ameliorate the fears or health problems from which the person is seeking relief. A reasonable initial approach would be to offer the guidelines presented in Table 12.1 and a consultation with a registered dietitian.

■ DIET AND NUTRITION FOR MEN WITH EARLY-STAGE PROSTATE CANCER AND SURVIVORS

A man with early-stage prostate cancer (organ confined) should receive an assessment of his nutritional status at the time of diagnosis, during the course of therapy, and periodically thereafter. A nutritional assessment coupled with a routine medical exam should include a diet and supplement history, simple anthropometric measurements, and a review of prescription and over-the-counter medications. This information, coupled with knowledge of the patient's other illnesses and past surgical procedures that are relevant to nutritional status, will guide the development of dietary and nutritional recommendations for each individual. Laboratory tests relevant to specific nutrients can be ordered for each patient, depending on the initial assessment and routine laboratory studies. It is unnecessary to routinely order measurements of nutritional markers, other than an initial screening for cholesterol and triglycerides, on all patients.

Men with newly diagnosed prostate cancer that is confined to the gland, based on physical exam and diagnostic testing, initially focus their attention on the treatment options with the hope of optimizing disease-free longevity with few complications of therapy. Once therapy has been defined, many patients and their families inquire about diet and nutritional recommendations that can improve outcome. There have been no studies that examine the effects of dietary intervention on the success of a local therapy such as prostatectomy, external beam radiation therapy, interstitial seed radiotherapy, or cryotherapy. Similarly, a role for nutritional intervention in men choosing observation has not been the subject of investigation. In the absence of well-defined studies, it is prudent to follow the guidelines provided in Table 12.1.

The period following initial therapy for prostate cancer is often when men and their families will fall prey to alternative health care practitioners, purveyors of nutrient supplements, and a host of other health promotion schemes (11,12,21). Victims of serious diseases such as prostate cancer, even those with a good prognosis, often feel desperate enough to try anything that offers hope of a better outcome. Quackery is often difficult to spot, even by physicians, and modern promoters use scientific jargon and effective sales pitches that can exploit the fears of prostate cancer patients. Alternative therapies that involve active participation by the patient can make a patient feel more in control of his outcome. Many men may also feel resentment toward the medical profession due to unexpected side effects of their prostate cancer therapy, such as impotence or incontinence. Although many Americans suffer harm to varying degrees, and certainly financial loss, due to quackery, few seem to consider it a serious problem. Many people are under the impression that government agencies offer enough sciuting to protect the public. However, laws regarding dietary supplements are weak and resources are not available for government agencies to investigate and prosecute purveyors of quackery. Physicians should be aware of these issues and provide patients with reasonable guidelines before they become unsuspecting victims of fraud.

Prostate cancer is a disease of older men, and many of the nutritional issues pertinent to the elderly should be considered in men with prostate cancer. As men age, there is a decline in the energy requirement secondary to reduced lean body mass. On average, daily calorie needs drop by about 10% each decade after age 50, but there is no significant decrease in the need for other nutrients. A decline in macronutrient intake because of reduced energy needs may contribute to an insufficient intake of various vitamins and minerals. Thus foods should be chosen more carefully to ensure adequate intake of nutrients, as there is less room for empty calories in the form of highly processed and refined foods. For example, many elderly persons can become overweight and undernourished through the consumption of sweets, cakes, and candy that are high in calories and low in nutrients. In addition, a number of other factors often contribute to poor nutrition in the elderly. These include economic factors, loss of mobility due to physical limitations, loss of means of transportation, concomitant conditions such as dentures, or illnesses such as neurologic problems or depression. All of these may lead to reduced access to food stores, decreased desire to shop, diminished desire to eat, or inability to eat properly.

As the American population has aged, there has been an increased awareness of the differences in the nutritional needs of the elderly (12). Research programs are beginning to define age-related physiologic and lifestyle changes that suggest unique nutrient requirements for the elderly. For example, some experts recommend that the current RDA for calcium of 800 mg/day should be increased to 1,000 or 1,500 mg to achieve calcium balance and good skeletal health. The recent dietary surveys of Americans over the age of 50 show that calcium intake for African-American men over the age of 60 and white men above the age of 70 are insufficient. The body's ability to use calcium properly requires vitamin D, the intake of which is also frequently marginal in the elderly. These data are consistent with a number of studies showing reduced consumption of vitamin D–fortified dairy products, which for some individuals is related to intolerance of dairy products. Older Americans also get less sunlight for vitamin D synthesis in the skin. Physicians should be aware of their patients' intake patterns relative to vitamin D and calcium and provide appropriate guidance.

Another nutrient that is frequently low in elderly men is iron. Supplementation may be necessary in the older population, due to poor diet and reduced intake of meat, particularly in those who have experienced increased blood loss for any reason. Some studies suggest that older people are also consuming insufficient zinc, a mineral needed for proper wound healing, metabolism, and immune function. Readily absorbable zinc is found in eggs and meats, particularly seafoods. Although zinc is found in many grains and other vegetables, its absorption may be compromised by high-fiber diets and natural substances that bind the mineral. Thus elderly vegetarians are at greater risk of deficiency.

Aging adults use almost 25% of the over-the-counter drugs sold in the United States, and the vast majority of elderly adults take at least one prescription drug daily. Physicians should be aware of some of the common nutrition and drug interactions (12). Drugs can depress appetite, alter taste or smell, and interfere with digestive processes. Some drugs contribute directly to nutrient loss. Common examples are aspirin and nonsteroidal anti-inflammatories (NSAIDs), which are frequently consumed on a chronic basis and may cause gastric blood loss, contributing to iron deficiency anemia. Chronic use of antacids can interfere with nutrient absorption. Laxatives, particularly mineral oil, can reduce absorption of fat-soluble vitamin D, A, K, and E. Physicians and elderly patients should be well informed about the medications consumed and their interactions with nutritional status.

■ DIET AND NUTRITION IN THE PATIENT WITH ADVANCED PROSTATE CANCER

Patients with metastatic prostate cancer are frequently affected by anorexia, decreased food intake, weight loss, and muscle wasting. These signs and symptoms are associated with increased fatigue and a progressive decline in overall functional status. This process is often referred to as the cancer cachexia syndrome. Although nutritional support alone will not significantly prolong survival, it may have a favorable impact on quality of life for many patients. Many factors contribute to the decline in nutritional status observed in advanced prostate cancer, including nausea; vomiting; early satiety; direct tumor encroachment on the gastrointestinal tract; iatrogenic causes, such as radiotherapy and anticancer agents; pain; and psychological distress (22). The wasting process frightens the patient and the family members, who frequently plead with caregivers for advice and interventions that will improve appetite and nutrition, to reverse the consumptive process in the hope that this will lead to a prolonged and better quality life.

Nutritional Assessment

A nutritional assessment of the patient with metastatic disease should include pre-illness weight, current weight, height, rate of weight loss, and presence of anorexia, dysphagia, nausea, vomiting, diarrhea, constipation, and associated problems. Ideal body weight should be calculated using standard tables and compared with actual weight. Laboratory parameters specifically designed to assess nutritional status are costly and should be requested only when an initial evaluation of the patient and routine chemistries and blood counts suggest that further studies are needed. All patients suffering from the cachexia syndrome or at risk of malnutrition should undergo evaluation by a clinical dietitian, who can quickly evaluate nutritional status and provide counseling appropriate for the individual situation.

Cancer Cachexia Syndrome

The cachexia syndrome in prostate cancer is characterized by worsening anorexia, progressive asthenia, relentless weight loss, and a progressive decline and derangement of various organ and tissue functions, which ultimately contribute to death. Cancer cachexia cannot be equated with starvation, which is how the process is often perceived by many family members. In starvation, metabolic efficiency increases and adipose tissue is lost while lean body mass and organ functions are preserved. In cancer cachexia, muscle and visceral protein is consumed, in addition to the body fat stores. In the presence of metastatic cancer, the body also continues to maintain a higher energy expenditure and relative inefficiency of metabolism, despite progressive anorexia. A number of metabolic and biochemical abnormalities are seen during cancer cachexia, including increased glucose turnover, relative insulin resistance, reduced protein and lipid synthesis, and wasted energy expenditure (22). With forced nutrition, a positive energy balance can be transiently achieved in some patients, but as the prostate cancer progresses, the metabolic perturbations increase. Ongoing efforts to understand the pathogenesis of cachexia may lead to the development of pharmacologic agents that can reverse some of the symptoms. Prostate tumors or host cells at metastatic sites probably secrete a number of factors that result in reduced appetite and alterations in the host metabolism. A number of growth factors or cytokines, such as TNF-α, IFN-γ, IL-1, IL-6, and others, may be involved.

Interventions

The cancer cachexia syndrome is a challenging clinical problem for the medical team. The most effective therapy for the wasting that occurs with prostate cancer would be the development of effective therapy for metastatic disease. Aggressive enteral and parenteral nutrition alone has not been shown to increase the life span of the cachectic prostate cancer patient. The dietary and nutritional interventions are therefore directed at improving the quality of life.

The physician is responsible for recognizing and aggressively treating the pain, nausea, constipation, and depression that can significantly contribute to reduced dietary intake. Anorexia is a key component of the cachexia syndrome and is associated with changes in smell and taste perception, food aversions, early satiety and nausea, problems with digestive and absorptive processes, and depression. Many of the interventions described below attempt to reverse or compensate for the anorexia component of the cachexia syndrome.

Counseling by a registered dietitian, preferably in the context of a team approach with the physician, primary nurse, and family, can improve patient satisfaction with care, improve or maintain nutritional status, relieve anxiety by providing guidelines and protocols, and prevent the patient and family from pursuing unproven, dangerous, and expensive alternative therapies. A number of empirical approaches may improve food consumption. For example, anorexia often progresses over the course of the day, and the patient can take advantage of a better morning appetite by having a more substantial breakfast. The patient should nibble frequently and drink commercially available liquid-nutrition preparations between meals. It is also very important that family members not make mealtime more stressful than necessary by forcing the patient to eat more than he wants.

Dietary supplements are an important component of nutritional support for many patients who are failing to obtain adequate nutrition through the diet but are able to swallow and have an intact gastrointestinal tract. These preparations are nutritionally balanced, easily digestible, and readily absorbed. The liquid concentrated food supplements provide a rich source of calories as well as protein, vitamins, and minerals. For patients who are not lactose intolerant, the use of "instant breakfast" mix with milk is an inexpensive and useful product. Commercial, premixed, ready-to-drink products are slightly more expensive and better tolerated in patients with lactose intolerance.

Appetite stimulants are being tested in clinical studies of cancer- and AIDS-associated anorexia and cachexia. Several drugs may have value in selected cases. These include corticosteroids, megestrol acetate, metoclopramide hydrochloride, and delta-9-tetrahydrocannabinol (THC). Corticosteroids are often used for their appetite-stimulating effects and to increase the patient's overall sense of well-being, although the optimal dosage and efficacy with regard to nutritional parameters have not been well established in controlled trials (22). A 4-mg dose of dexamethasone every morning following breakfast is a reasonable initial approach. If no response is observed, a second dose of 4 mg with lunch can be included. The timing is important, since evening dosing is associated with insomnia. Dexamethasone is contraindicated in diabetic patients and should be stopped if proximal myopathy, fluid retention, or mental status changes are seen. Agents such as ranitidine hydrochloride are frequently used to prevent gastrointestinal intolerance. Metoclopramide hydrochloride may be useful in patients with early satiety and nausea associated with delayed upper gastrointestinal motility. Physicians should consider a trial of metoclopramide in those having opioid-induced dysmotility, although clinical studies in this subpopulation have not been completed. A dose of 10 mg before meals and at bedtime is usually effective. Metoclopramide is contraindicated in patients with dyskinetic disorders, and dose reductions may be necessary due to dystonic reactions or a sense of hyperactivity. Megestrol acetate has been used for the hormonal therapy of breast cancer for many years and has been found to produce weight gain, increased appetite, and improved overall sense of well-being (22,23). A randomized, double-blind, placebo-controlled study of megestrol acetate in patients with advanced cancer showed significant improvements in appetite, food intake, nausea, and emesis (23). It is reasonable to start at a dose of 160 mg/day, which is well tolerated in patients with advanced cancer and relatively poor performance status. However, patients with a history of deep venous thrombosis, congestive heart failure, or diabetes should not use megestrol acetate. The most common side effects at this dosage are peripheral edema, mild hyperglycemia, and a decline in sexual function. Additional studies of megestrol acetate in prostate cancer patients are needed to define optimal dose and efficacy. Studies of THC as an antiemetic for cancer chemotherapy revealed overall improvement in appetite. A role for THC in men with advanced prostate cancer has not been carefully evaluated. A dose of 2.5 mg with breakfast and lunch is a reasonable initial regimen to assess patient response and side effects. An additional dose with the evening meal can be added. THC may be most useful in those with a mild depression not requiring antidepressants, but it should be avoided in those with preexisting cognitive and psychological problems. The major side effects of THC are euphoria, somnolence, dizziness, and confusion.

It is rare that a prostate cancer patient will benefit from enteral alimentation or parenteral nutrition. Enteral nutrition using a nasogastric, gastrostomy, or jejunostomy tube is indicated only in those who are unable to swallow or who have obstructions or a dysfunction that prevents the safe ingestion of food into the upper gastrointestinal tract. The risks of enteral feeding include aspiration, diarrhea, nausea, vomiting, cramps, bloating, and distention. Prostate cancer patients who are unable to achieve their nutritional needs via the enteral route and who have a complication of their disease that is treatable by surgery, radiation, or drug therapy—and who, in addition, have a reasonable life expectancy—may be candidates for total parenteral nutrition. Very few patients with advanced prostate cancer meet these criteria. Complications associated with total parenteral nutrition include catheter-related pneumothorax, infection, thrombosis, hepatic dysfunction, and fluid and electrolyte imbalance. There are no studies suggesting that aggressive enteral or parenteral feeding reverses the cancer cachexia syndrome, improves quality of life, or prolongs survival in most patients with advanced prostate cancer. Many issues should be carefully evaluated when enteral or parenteral nutrition is considered. Ethical issues, the wishes of the patient and family, expense, necessity of additional human and laboratory support, and clinical circumstances must be carefully balanced in order to make appropriate decisions.

Editorial Comment

The role of diet and nutrition in prostate cancer prevention and therapy has been a neglected area of investigation. Although much more needs to be learned through epidemiologic and laboratory studies, the public is seeking information concerning dietary and nutritional recommendations to prevent prostate cancer and other diseases of aging. It appears that a shift away from the typical diet found in affluent nations may provide some protection from prostate cancer. A dietary pattern which is lower in energy, fat, animal products, and higher in fruits, vegetables, and fiber is a reasonable approach for prostate cancer prevention. However, it is not known whether such a diet must be lifelong in order to provide such a benefit. It is also unknown at the present time whether diet adjustment after the diagnosis of prostate cancer can have an impact on disease progression and patient survival.

Patients should be aware that the lay literature will always be flooded with new dietary "supplements" to shrink the prostate or cure prostate cancer. The patient must read such literature critically and should consult his physicians and his local chapter of the American Cancer Society for help in distinguishing fact from fantasy.

■ REFERENCES

1. Boring CC, Squires TS, Heath CW, et al. Cancer statistics for African Americans. CA 1992;42:7–18.
2. Boring CC, Squires TS, Tong T, et al. Cancer statistics. CA 1994;44:7–26.
3. Whittemore AS, Kolonel LN, Wu AH, et al. Prostate cancer in relation to diet, physical activity, and body size in blacks, whites, and Asians in the United States and Canada. J Natl Cancer Inst 1995;87:652–661.
4. Clinton SK. Nutrition in the etiology and prevention of cancer. In: Holland JA, Frei E, Bast RC, et al., eds. Cancer Medicine. Philadelphia: Lea and Febiger, 1993.
5. Pienta KJ, Espar PS. Risk factors for prostate cancer. Ann Intern Med 1993;118:793–803.
6. National Research Council of the National Academy of Sciences. Diet, nutrition, and cancer. Washington, DC: National Academy Press, 1982.
7. National Cancer Institute. Diet, nutrition, and cancer prevention: a guide to food choices. NIH Pub. No. 87-28-78. National Institutes of Health, Public Health Service, US Department of Health and Human Services. Washington, DC: US Government Printing Office, 1987.
8. National Research Council of the National Academy of Sciences. Diet and health. Washington, DC: National Academy Press, 1989.
9. World Health Organization. Diet, nutrition and the prevention of chronic diseases. Technical Report Series, No. 797. Geneva: World Health Organization, 1990.
10. American Cancer Society. Guidelines on diet, nutrition, and cancer. CA 1991;41:334.
11. Barrett S, Herbert V. The vitamin pushers. Amherst, New York: Prometheus Books, 1994.

12. Herbert V, Subak-Sharpe GJ. Total nutrition: the only guide you'll ever need. New York: St. Martin's Press, 1995.

13. Albanes D. Total calories, body weight, and tumor incidence in mice. Cancer Res 1987;47:1987–1992.

14. Clinton, SK, Giovannucci E. Nutrition in the etiology and prevention of cancer. In Holland JA, Frei E, Bast RC, et al. (eds). Cancer Medicine. Philadelphia, Lea and Febiger, 1996.

15. Giovannucci E, Rimm EB, Colditz GA, et al. A prospective study of dietary fat and risk of prostate cancer. J Natl Cancer Inst 1993;85:1571–1579.

16. Giovannucci E, Rimm EB, Stampfer MJ, et al. Intake of fat, meat, and fiber in relation to risk of colon cancer in men. Cancer Res 1994;2390–2397.

17. Wang Y, Corr JG, Thaler HT, et al. Decreased growth of established human prostate LNCaP tumors in nude mice fed a low-fat diet. J Natl Cancer Inst 1995;87:1456–1462.

18. Block G, Patterson B, Subar A, et al. Fruit, vegetables, and cancer prevention: a review of the epidemiological evidence. Nutr Cancer 1992;18:1–29.

19. Giovannucci EL, Ascherio A, Rimm EB, et al. Intake of carotenoids and retinol in relationship to risk of prostate cancer. J Natl Cancer Inst 1995;87:1767–1776.

20. Clinton SK, Emenhiser C, Schwartz SJ, et al. Cis-translycopene isomers, carotenoids, and retinol in the human prostate. In: Cancer epidemiology, biomarkers, and prevention. Cancer Epidemiology, Biomarkers, and Prevention. 1996;5:823–833.

21. Zwicky JF, Hafner AW, Barrett S, et al. Reader's guide to alternative health methods. Chicago: American Medical Association, 1993.

22. Nelson KA, Walsh D, Sheehan FA, et al. The cancer anorexia-cachexia syndrome. J Clin Oncol 1994;12:213–225.

23. Loprinzi CL, Ellison NM, Schaid D, et al. Controlled trial of megestrol acetate for the treatment of cancer anorexia and cachexia. J Natl Cancer Inst 1990;82:1127–1132.

Index

▼ ▼ ▼ ▼ ▼ ▼ ▼ ▼